The EVERYTHING. Easy Fitness Book

Dear Reader,

Years ago, when I was in my early twenties, I walked about seven miles a day (including hill climbing), took aerobics and yoga classes, and swam every morning. I was always tired. I never ate (I very mistakenly thought I was fat), and I was always in a bad mood (hunger and exhaustion will do that to you).

Now, twenty years later, I weigh a fair amount more than I used to, and I exercise more sanely. I walk the dog, I do yoga, I ice skate with my son, and I lift weights a few times a week. I eat. I am almost always in a good mood, and I feel good about myself. I'm no longer obsessed with exercise, even though it is my second favorite thing to do (the first is take care of my son).

To me, easy fitness means livable fitness. It means making sure that your life is balanced and that you are happy with the activity and the activity level you have in your life. It doesn't mean being a slave to the idea of being thin or athletic or a certain size clothing. Fitness doesn't have to mean accomplishing a series of athletic skills, but can instead be the way you live your life as a strong, flexible, and physically capable person.

What I hope, most of all, is that this book makes you want to go outside and take a walk, or play soccer with your kids, or go swimming on a Saturday afternoon. Your body loves to move, it wants to move, and when it moves, it naturally becomes fit. That's how easy it is.

Best wishes,

Donna Raskin

The EVERYTHING® Series

Editorial

Publishing Director	Gary M. Krebs
Director of Product Development	Paula Munier
Associate Managing Editor	Laura M. Daly
Associate Copy Chief	Brett Palana-Shanahan
Acquisitions Editor	Lisa Laing
Development Editor	Katie McDonough
Associate Production Editor	Casey Ebert

Production

Director of Manufacturing	Susan Beale
Associate Director of Production	Michelle Roy Kelly
Cover Design	Paul Beatrice Matt LeBlanc Erick DaCosta
Design and Layout	Heather Barrett Brewster Brownville Colleen Cunningham Jennifer Oliveira
Series Cover Artist	Barry Littmann

Visit the entire Everything® Series at *www.everything.com*

THE
EVERYTHING®
EASY FITNESS
BOOK
2nd Edition

Lose weight, build strength, and feel energized

Donna Raskin

Adams Media
Avon, Massachusetts

This book is dedicated to my brothers and sisters: Peter, Danielle, Angelo, and Morgan,
and my sister-in-law and nephew, Paula and Dylan. I love you all, and even though I have
lived far away for many years, you are all always in my thoughts and in my heart.

An Everything® Series Book.
Everything® and everything.com® are registered trademarks of F+W Publications, Inc.

Published by Adams Media, an F+W Publications Company
57 Littlefield Street, Avon, MA 02322 U.S.A.
www.adamsmedia.com

ISBN 10: 1-59337-699-5
ISBN 13: 978-1-59337-699-4

Printed in the United States of America.

J   I   H   G   F   E   D   C   B

Library of Congress Cataloging-in-Publication Data

Raskin, Donna.
The everything easy fitness book / Donna Raskin. -- 2nd ed.
p. cm. -- (Everything series)
Includes index.
ISBN-13: 978-1-59337-699-4
ISBN-10: 1-59337-699-5
1. Physical fitness. 2. Exercise. I. Title.

RA781.R27 2006
613.7--dc22
2006028192

Disclaimer: The exercise program within The Everything® Wedding Workout Book or any other exercise program may result in injury. Consult your doctor before beginning this or any exercise program. If you begin to feel faint or dizzy while doing any of the exercises in this book, consult your doctor.

This publication is designed to provide accurate and authoritative information with regard to the subject matter covered. It is sold with the understanding that the publisher is not engaged in rendering legal, accounting, or other professional advice. If legal advice or other expert assistance is required, the services of a competent professional person should be sought.

—From a *Declaration of Principles* jointly adopted by a Committee of the
American Bar Association and a Committee of Publishers and Associations

Many of the designations used by manufacturers and sellers to distinguish their products are claimed as trademarks. Where those designations appear in this book and Adams Media was aware of a trademark claim, the designations have been printed with initial capital letters.

This book is available at quantity discounts for bulk purchases.
For information, please call 1-800-289-0963.

Interior illustrations by Mark Divico

Contents

Acknowledgments

Thank you to Paula Munier for her friendship, support, laughter, and publishing expertise. I want to thank Lisa Laing for her patience, and for laughing when she could have been frustrated. That's a rare gift, and I appreciate it. Thank you to Laura Daly for her ability to alter schedules when necessary (a powerful gift), and to Andrea Norville for her support with this project.

Top Ten Benefits of Easy Fitness

1. You will feel strong and energetic, but you won't look bulky or unnatural.

2. You will learn how to burn more calories and fat during your workouts.

3. You will create long, lean muscles that help you feel graceful and elegant.

4. You will want to move more than you'll want to sit on the couch and watch TV.

5. If you work in an office, you will learn how to make your day energizing, rather than exhausting.

6. If you have small children, you will learn how to make sure they are active, too.

7. You will learn how to eat for health and fitness. Of course you're going to eat chocolate! It's good for you!

8. You will learn how to work with your body as it ages, rather than giving in to the false belief that the body has to disintegrate as you get older.

9. You will find balance in your life, and it will include activity and rest, and high-intensity movement and relaxing movement.

10. You will look in the mirror and like what you see.

Introduction

▶ EASY FITNESS DOESN'T MEAN following a regimented work-out program or dedicating your entire life to exercise. Easy fitness means being active, creating and sticking to regular exercise times in your schedule, and eating well and sleeping enough so that your body is able to thrive, not just survive.

Exercise doesn't have to be difficult or complicated to be effective. While it's certainly true that athletes and people who love to work out often have complicated workout programs, *you* don't have to complicate exercise. You can get into shape just by doing the things you like to do and having a small amount of knowledge about how to turn your likes—whether they are walking, gardening, or dancing—into an exercise routine that will not only keep you healthy, but also fit.

So, what is the difference between health and fitness? The following comparison will illustrate the distinction. In the first scenario it's 7:00 A.M. on Thanksgiving morning. A forty-two-year-old woman is putting a turkey in the oven. She is on her feet in the kitchen most of the morning, and then spends much of the afternoon going from the table to the kitchen, serving her family and friends. In the evening, she washes dishes, cleans the house, does a load of laundry, and finally gets a chance to eat some of her pumpkin pie while she watches TV. The day was tiring, but she had fun. She wasn't exhausted at the end, she ate well (maybe a little too much stuffing and spinach dip), and she slept well that night. She is exhausted the next day, and instead of going shopping as she had planned, she spends most of the day on her couch. She has to take a pain reliever to soothe the aches and pains she feels, and even though she was completely full after the meal the day before, she ends up eating two slices of pie and the rest of the sweet potatoes. By Saturday, though, she's fine and at the mall. She is healthy.

Now, picture another forty-two-year-old woman. She is also celebrating Thanksgiving. Nevertheless, she starts her day the same way she starts every other day, with a 10-minute yoga routine. She likes yoga because she doesn't even have to get out of her pajamas to do it. She cooks all morning, but takes a 20-minute break to play touch football with her fifteen-year-old just before she jumps in the shower. After all of the eating (she also enjoyed the stuffing but abstained from the spinach dip), she takes a walk around the block with her husband. The day went well. She sleeps great all night, and when she wakes up she heads straight to the gym for her three-times-a-week burn-and-sculpt exercise class. She hasn't gained any weight in the last eight years, and she can still do every move she learned when she was thirty-four. This woman is fit.

Being fit is more than being healthy. In the most obvious and simple definition, being fit means you have energy, are active (not sedentary), are strong, have a healthy heart, are flexible, and are the proper weight. For the purposes of this book, fitness is functional, not athletic.

An easy fitness week has a few elements. First, there have to be a few scheduled workout sessions that get your heart pumping, increase your muscular strength and endurance, and increase your flexibility and balance. These workouts will be focused and have a purpose so that you will see a difference in how you look and how you feel. Second, there have to be times when you choose to do fun things that are active rather than sedentary. So, for example, you'll go for a walk after dinner rather than watching TV. Or you'll choose to play a game of tetherball with your kids rather than sitting next to the pool while they play.

The third element of your easy fitness week will be creating a system that supports your fitness plans. This will include eating well, getting enough rest, having friends around who will help if you need it, and, most importantly, reading this book, which will give you all the information and support you need to create your new fit life.

Chapter 1
Fitness and Exercise

Exercise keeps our bodies and all of their parts working efficiently. When your heart is fit, it beats more strongly but uses less energy to keep pumping. When your muscles are fit, they can lift more and work longer without feeling stress or getting hurt. When your entire body is fit, you burn more calories, sleep better at night, and have a stronger immune system. When you exercise regularly and effectively, your body is lean, sleek, and capable. A fit body takes up less room than an unfit body, but it is able to do far more.

The Elements of Fitness

You know fitness when you see it—a strong body, thin and thriving. You see someone who bounds up the stairs, who stretches easily without straining or grasping his lower back, and you consider him fit. You watch a woman dance without having to catch her breath or sit down, and you believe she is fit. You see a man play football with his son and think "fit."

Fitness sometimes seems like a gift—you either have it or you don't. But in reality, fitness is something you create. To become fit and create a fit life, you need to know what healthy traits and habits compose fitness and how you can go about improving your levels of them. Once you know those things—and once you make their practice a regular part of your life—you will be fit. Fitness is composed of cardiorespiratory health, muscle strength and endurance, and flexibility.

Cardiorespiratory Health

The heart is a muscle that pumps blood through the body via the vascular system, which is composed of your veins and arteries. Meanwhile, your lungs extract oxygen from the air you breathe and send it into the blood for distribution throughout the body.

Heart and lung health, or cardiorespiratory health, means your heart, lungs, and vascular system work together to efficiently process and transport oxygen to your muscles. When your heart is strong, it easily pumps more blood throughout your body. When your heart is weak, it takes more work for it to provide your body with fresh blood and oxygen. If your heart and lungs aren't strong, then even light physical activity, such as carrying a bag of groceries from the car to the house, or walking a little faster around the block, can leave you out of breath.

Muscle Strength and Endurance

Muscle strength means how much weight a muscle can lift, while muscle endurance means how long a muscle can work lifting various weight amounts. Strength is relative. For example, if a twenty-five-year-old man can't lift his five-year-old daughter, he would be considered weak. If his seventy-year-old grandmother can lift the five-year-old, then she's doing pretty well, strength-wise.

Strong muscles are able to lift a very heavy weight once or twice, and a moderate weight more often or for longer periods of time. Putting grocery bags in your car and carrying them to your house illustrate muscle strength and muscle endurance. Let's say you have two heavy grocery bags, and you can lift them from your shopping cart and put them into your car. That's strength. And even if the bags are moderately heavy, you can probably carry them from the trunk of your car parked in your garage to your house fifty feet away. That's muscle endurance.

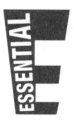

Weight-resistance exercise also improves bone health because muscle attaches to bone. Stronger bones help stave off osteoporosis and other debilitating diseases. When your bones are strong, you stand straight, breathe more deeply, and are less like to get injured, especially as you age.

Flexibility

Flexibility is the ability to move a joint throughout its range of motion. A joint is the place where two or more bones meet; bones are connected by ligaments and tendons, which are connective tissues. Joints allow movement in the body, and flexibility is necessary for efficient movement. Being flexible may also decrease the chance of sustaining muscular injury, soreness, and pain. In other words, when a person lacks flexibility, movement can be limiting, painful, and disabling. Flexibility is essential to your health and a valuable component of your exercise program.

Flexibility exercises are those that gently stretch muscles, tendons, and ligaments to keep them pliable and mobile. Flexibility exercises include stretching, ballet, yoga, and tai chi. When you are fit and flexible, your body is able to do more with less effort, and that feels great and encourages more activity.

Aerobic Versus Anaerobic Exercise

To make the heart stronger, you need to train it to pump blood more efficiently throughout the body. This training is done through aerobic exercise. Aerobic exercise makes you breathe more heavily than you usually do because you are using oxygen more rapidly since your body is moving faster than usual. Aerobic exercise strengthens the heart, blood vessels, and lungs by training them to process and carry blood and oxygen faster and more powerfully. An activity is usually aerobic when you move several of your limbs at the same time, and when the activity uses the big muscle groups (for example, the hips, legs, chest, and back). The activity must be performed continuously (more than 20 minutes), is usually rhythmic or repetitive, and is performed at an intensity level that causes your heart, lungs, and vascular system to work harder than usual. For example, turning a stroll into a fast walk, turning splashing in the pool into a five-lap race, or turning a neighborhood bike ride into a spinning class are all examples of regular activity becoming aerobic activity.

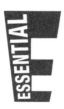

When you exercise aerobically, you take in greater amounts of oxygen and deliver it more deeply in the body. The body loves regular bouts of oxygen-rich exercise, and the benefits appear not only during exercise but also while the body is at rest.

One intensity level above and beyond aerobic exercise is anaerobic exercise. To make great strides in cardiovascular health, you can use anaerobic exercise intermittently during your exercise session to overload the cardiovascular system. You can't sustain anaerobic exercise for very long. It's comparable to a sprint—you work as hard and as fast as you can for less than a minute. These intervals of high-intensity exercise expand and increase your aerobic capacity by pushing you past your aerobic limits. Then when you go back to your previous aerobic levels, your heart will be stronger, and the work will feel easier.

The Overload Principle

Aerobic and anaerobic exercise use the overload principle for training. The overload principle states that to improve your fitness, you need to work your body harder than it is used to working. Research has found that your body adapts to the stress of working harder by becoming stronger. For example, if you walk two miles fives days a week, eventually walking those two miles will get easier, and you'll be able to work longer or faster or both. Your heart becomes stronger and more efficient using the overload principle, but you can apply this principle to the other components of physical fitness, including muscle strength, muscle endurance, and flexibility.

Muscles and Overload

By systematically overloading your muscles in both strength and endurance (lifting more weight or lifting weight for longer), as well as in flexibility (stretching further and more extensively) you will also be able to make gains in those fitness elements. Lifting weights and stretching in a regular strengthening program allows you to create a body that is more capable and fitter than it was before.

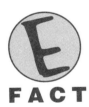

FACT

The American College of Sports Medicine (ACSM) is the largest sports medicine and exercise-science organization in the world, with over 15,000 members in more than seventy-two countries. ACSM members include doctors, educators, scientists, personal trainers, group-exercise instructors, and other health and fitness professionals. The recommendations in this book follow ACSM guidelines.

Your fitness level determines how much overload you will use when you exercise. If you have been sedentary, here is some good news: it won't take much to overload your heart and other muscles, so your fitness will improve quickly. If you have been exercising for a while but haven't seen improvements, it may be due to a lack of overload in your activity. So once you start working harder, you'll see improvements, too.

FITT and Overload

To properly incorporate the overload principle into your fitness routine, you can rely on FITT. FITT is an acronym for the four elements that make up an effective exercise program:

Frequency—how often you exercise
Intensity—how hard you exercise
Time—how long you exercise
Type—mode or type of exercise

Frequency, Intensity, Time, and Type of Exercise

As mentioned previously, frequency refers to how often you exercise. You'll need to do 30 minutes of moderate activity daily (which can be broken up into 10-minute sessions) to stay healthy, and three or four high-intensity workouts each week to stay truly fit. The more you exercise, the more calories you burn, and the stronger your heart and muscles are.

Keeping the overload principle in mind, you'll need to be aware of your intensity level to make sure you are working hard enough to overload your heart and your muscles while you exercise. Moderate-intensity exercise gets your heart pumping, but not in an overly stressful, breathless way. This kind of exercise helps you develop endurance. High-intensity exercise is tough; you breathe heavily and are overloading your heart and muscles. You need a mixture of both kinds of intensity to stay fit. When you push your intensity levels, your body responds by becoming stronger and burning more calories.

How long are you working out? Is it enough to build endurance and allow for proper overloading? The more time you spend exercising, the greater the results in terms of strength and endurance.

The fittest bodies and healthiest people get that way due to a variety of types of exercises, such as walking, weightlifting, and yoga; or bicycling, swimming, and gardening. The more variety in your exercise program, the more likely it is that your body will increase its strength, endurance, and flexibility—and the less likely it is that you'll suffer from overuse injuries.

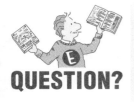

QUESTION?

What is the difference between moderate-intensity and high-intensity exercise?

Intensity refers to how hard your heart and muscles are working during a given activity. In practical terms, a stroll is low intensity, a brisk walk is moderate intensity, and a fast walk/jog program is high intensity. Likewise, playing in the pool is low intensity, swimming laps is moderate intensity, and racing is high intensity. To provide one last example, gardening on your knees is low intensity, raking is moderate intensity, and moving shrubs and young trees is high intensity.

Adding Intensity to Your Workouts

As you read, the "I" in FITT stands for intensity, or as explained previously, how hard you are working. Intensity can refer to your heart, your muscles, or your entire body as a whole. The more intensely you exercise, the more you will be applying the overload principle. However, you can't just push your body to an extreme limit right away. If you do that, you'll get hurt and end up not seeing any benefits. Instead, when you exercise, you need to increase the intensity gradually so that your body gets fitter over time.

There are several ways to add intensity to your workouts. You can, for example, add runs to your walk, or lift heavier weights, or add another activity or exercise session to your routine. But to increase intensity, you have to know how to measure it. It's impossible to make your workouts tougher if you aren't sure how hard they are to begin with.

Intensity Levels

ACSM recommends that you exercise at aerobic intensity levels of 60 to 90 percent of your maximum heart rate. Your goal is to match up your current level of fitness with the appropriate intensity levels in your exercise program. If you are just starting to exercise, you will begin exercising so that your heart rate stays around 60 percent of its maximum. Once your body has adapted to that level, you can then progress slowly and gradually into higher levels of intensity, which will also help you burn fat more efficiently.

While exercising at 60 percent of your maximum heart rate may seem to require very light effort, this still benefits your cardiovascular system by training it to work more efficiently without overstressing it. Exercising at an aerobic level of 85 percent of your maximum heart rate requires more effort, but in the beginning you can only stay at that level for a short amount of time.

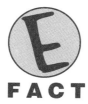

FACT

Exercise increases endorphin production. Endorphins are natural morphine-like hormones that produce a sense of well-being, and that reduce stress. Regular exercise triggers their release. The effect of endorphins can last for hours or even a few days, but beyond that, you have to reproduce them.

In the past, beginning exercisers were told that they would burn more fat if they exercised at a lower intensity, because it was known that the body uses glucose, a sugar in the blood, for fuel when it exercises more intensely. However, the truth is, the harder you exercise, the higher levels of both fat and sugar you'll burn. If you want to lose weight and burn off fat, you'll need to gradually work your way up to more intense levels of exercise. You'll read more about how to do that in Chapter 2.

Intensity and Calorie-burning

Your body is working all the time: pumping blood, processing food, thinking. The body's unit of measurement for the amount of work it's doing is called the calorie. When you sit and think, you burn about one calorie per minute. When you take a walk, your body might burn from three to six calories a minute. For every one liter of oxygen (per kilogram of body weight) you process during aerobic exercise, the body burns five calories. The more energy you use, the more oxygen you process, and the more calories you burn. Ideally, you should burn 300 calories or more per exercise session.

Your body's calorie usage during any given activity is determined by your weight, your fitness level, and the amount of work you're doing. Because of the difference in the muscle/fat ratio of their bodies, as well as their fitness levels, a slight, older woman burns fewer calories taking a walk than a young, muscular man.

Your heart rate, or pulse, reflects how hard your body and your heart are working at any given time. Your pulse, which is measured in beats per minute (bpm), is slow when you're asleep, faster when you're awake, and really fast when you work out hard.

Monitoring Your Heart Rate

Exercising without knowing your heart rate is the equivalent of driving without a speedometer. If you know your heart rate, you know how hard you are working. Knowing your heart rate makes you more productive and efficient during your exercise time if you also know how much your heart rate should be for you to be burning the right amount of calories. The most exact way to gauge exercise intensity is to use a heart-rate monitor, but you can also take your pulse to determine how hard your heart is working.

Measure Your Pulse

You can measure your pulse by using your fingers at your carotid (neck) artery or the radial (wrist) artery. The carotid pulse is located just below the top of the jaw, high up on either side of the neck. To feel it, put your first two fingers (not your thumb) lightly on this area. Exerting too much pressure can slow the heart rate, so touch this area gently. You should feel your pulse against your fingers.

The radial pulse can be found on the thumb side of the forearm just slightly above where the wrist naturally flexes and bends. As with the carotid pulse, use your first two fingers, not your thumb, to feel your pulse.

Count the beats for 15 seconds and multiply by four to estimate the number of beats per minute. Or count the beats for 10 seconds and multiply by six to estimate the number of beats per minute. Then compare this number in beats per minute (bpm) to your desired training zone. While you're estimating your pulse per minute here, this method is usually good enough to determine how hard you're working during exercise. Later in this chapter you will learn about what your target heart rate should be during exercise.

Using a Heart-rate Monitor

Heart-rate monitors have revolutionized aerobic fitness because they quickly and easily give you reliable information on how hard you are working. Typically, the monitor has two parts: a strap that goes around your chest (near your bra strap), and a device that you wear around your wrist, like a watch. The strap electronically monitors how fast your heart is beating and transmits the signal to the watch. Then you read the watch to find out how hard you're working. Heart-rate monitors cost about $100 and are well worth the price.

Before you use a heart-rate monitor, moisten the underside of the battery/sensor strap with water or saliva. The moisture helps conduct the electrical activity to the monitor. Then hold the strap against the front of your torso just below the breast area. Adjust the circumference of the elastic strap so that it is snug but not uncomfortable. Hold up the wrist monitor approximately 6 to 10 inches directly in front of the position of one of the sensors on the battery/sensor strap. This engages the communication between the sensors and the wrist monitor, and in a few moments your heart rate in beats per minute should be visible.

The monitor will read and display your heart rate in beats per minute as long as it stays within 1 to 3 feet of the sensors. Should you lose the signal in the middle of an exercise session, simply bring the wrist monitor up in front of the sensors again, and the monitor will re-engage. Bicyclists (stationary or regular) can mount the wrist monitor on their handlebars by using a bike-mount apparatus or by tightening the wrist strap around the bars.

Heart-rate Zone

To figure out what your heart rate or pulse should be when you exercise, use this (very rough) formula:

1. Subtract your age from 220. For example: If you are 40 years old, then the answer is 180. This number is your estimated maximum heart rate in beats per minute.
2. Now, multiply that number (e.g., 180) by .65 and .85. The two numbers (117 and 153) tell you the range your heart rate should be during exercise.

You will spend the majority of your exercise time with your heart rate in the lower part of the range, and will reach the higher part of the range only during brief interval sessions, which you will learn more about in Chapter 2. If you're very fit, you can use a slightly different formula to determine the range of your heart rate during exercise. As a first step, subtract your age from 205, and then do the rest of the calculations as they have been described previously.

Rating of Perceived Exertion

Another less scientific yet helpful way to gauge exercise intensity is the Borg scale for Rating of Perceived Exertion, more commonly known as RPE. The key word here is *perceived* because you are using your own sense of your body to gauge how hard you are working. Therefore, this is a subjective measure of how hard you are exercising. The Borg scale goes from 6 to 19.

Amazingly, Borg found that if you add a zero to the number of your perceived exertion, you would very often be working at that heart rate. So, for example, if you feel as if you're working at level 14, chances are your heart rate is somewhere around 140.

6–7	Very, very light
8–9	Very light
10–11	Fairly light
12–13	Somewhat hard
14–15	Hard
16–17	Very hard
18–19	Very, very hard

The Pros of RPE

Despite the RPE's unscientific qualities, research has found that the scale corresponds consistently to the heart rate that a person experiences during exercise. For example, you are most likely to achieve the cardiorespiratory training effect at intensity levels that are "somewhat hard" to "hard" and these intensities correspond almost exactly to a rating of 12 to 15 on the scale.

Using Perception Properly

The con to the RPE is that it is, as mentioned, not scientific, and therefore inexact. But whatever your health, exercise level, or activity, your sense of intensity needs to be consistent. The Rate of Perceived Exertion scale uses your own sense of intensity to allow you to judge how hard you are working, but how hard is hard? You need to honestly evaluate how hard you are working, so here are some guidelines on how hard "hard" is (and how easy "easy" can be).

The first few numbers on the scale use the word "light," which means your heart is not pumping harder than it usually does when you walk around your house. "Somewhat hard" refers to the awareness that you are beginning to move with a specific intensity. You could keep going for a while and you aren't stressed, but you notice the movement. "Hard" is intense, and an activity level that could not be continued indefinitely. As it gets more intense, i.e., you're using the word "very," you would be less likely to be able to keep moving at that level for any length of time.

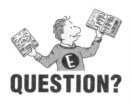

QUESTION?

What does "intense" feel like?

Lance Armstrong bikes a hundred miles and barely breaks a sweat. You might walk around the block and feel like you need to sit down for the next two hours. Intensity is very much a personal thing, based on your fitness level, age, the activity you're doing, and how you feel on that particular day.

Don't think about these specific words too deeply. The fact is, you know when you're working or not working. If you don't know, if you really can't feel how hard your body is working, then here are some questions to ask yourself, and the intensity levels your answers may correspond to.

Statement	Intensity	Equivalent
Wow, even though I'm walking I can count the spots on that ladybug.	6–7	Very, very light
This walk feels nice. I could do this for hours.	7–8	Very light
I think I'm walking faster than usually do.	9–11	Fairly light
My heart feels energized.	12–13	Somewhat hard
I'm breathing heavy. I'm glad I don't have to talk to anyone right now.	14–15	Hard
Soon I'm going to have to slow down.	16–17	Very hard
I have to stop.	18–19	Very, very hard

To use RPE, all you need to do is ask yourself periodically throughout your workout is: "How hard am I working?" Then answer honestly using the scale. If you find yourself not working hard enough, pick up your pace. If you're working too hard, slow down. It's that easy.

Chapter 2

Creating an Active Life

Imagine yourself walking briskly through the park, or dancing with someone you love, or biking on a sunny day. Visualize the elegant way you will move through your yoga routine, or how wonderful it will feel to do ten pushups or gracefully lift something into the trunk of your car. Now you will learn how to not only make your body active, but also let your mind come along for the ride. Easy fitness means you need to find workable, doable changes that will bring fitness into your life. This book will help you do it.

What You Need

To change the way you live your life, you need three things. First, you need to know what kind of change you want to make. To help you here, in this chapter you will learn more about what type of activity you need to incorporate into your life to see benefits. Next, you need the intention to change. To help you with that, in this chapter you will learn how to create active intentions, which will outline how you will add fitness into your life. Finally, you need a realistic plan for making change happen. Again, this chapter will show you how to do this. At the end of this chapter, you will have all of the tools you need to create an easy fitness plan that will enable you to reach your goals.

Activity in Your Life

To really be fit, you're going to have to find room for two things: (1) regular workouts that will strengthen your heart and other muscles, and that will burn calories; and (2) more activity in your day-to-day schedule, such as short walks and regular stretches. These two aspects of fitness cannot replace each other. You need both of them to truly be both healthy and fit.

The 30 minutes of daily activity can be of moderate intensity, which is the equivalent of walking 3.5 miles per hour. But the exercise sessions that you need for fitness and weight management need to include aerobic and anaerobic exercise for your heart, as well as strength training and flexibility sessions to keep your muscles strong and limber.

Making Activity Easy

For the purposes of this book, "easy" activity means nonstressful, workable ways to add exercise into your life. "Easy" means you can make your desk job more active, find time to go to the gym if you want to, create effective exercise sessions for your home, and take walks that burn fat and calories right off. Start your workout plans with activities you enjoy, whether they are biking, swimming, walking, or meditation. If you start with things you like to do, your goals will be that much easier to reach.

It won't be hard for you to adapt these changes to your life or for you to incorporate the changes into your schedule. Fitness is easy when it's fun and when you see results, and that doesn't mean you have to stick to a plan you don't enjoy, or do exercises that you hate. Instead, this plan is easy because you're going to like it.

Another part of your easy-fitness week is being active when previously you were sedentary. So for instance, you'll add a little yoga to your morning routine, or some dancing to your weekend plans, or you'll walk around the mall two times fast instead of sitting in the food court.

Your Fitness Schedule

In order to add more activity into your life, you'll need to schedule your workouts and always make sure your workouts count. You're not going to have to rearrange your entire life to be fit. But the reality is, if you don't schedule your workouts, you probably won't ever get around to exercising or being active. Therefore, you will need to schedule at least three, and hopefully four, 40-minute workout sessions into your week. But don't groan yet! The good news is that you choose what you'll do during those workouts. So take out your planner or your calendar, or even a blank piece of paper or a napkin, and write down when you're going to exercise.

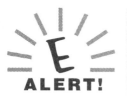

ALERT!

Don't limit yourself when scheduling your workouts. Be honest about how much time it actually takes you to get ready, travel to the facility (if you're using one), work out, and return home. If you have to drive to the gym or change clothes, then give yourself an hour even if you're only planning to exercise for 40 minutes. The last thing you want is to feel rushed by your own schedule.

In Chapter 1, you learned a little bit about how to make your workouts count by using the overload principle and FITT. In the following sections, you'll learn more about interval workouts, which turn fast workouts into powerhouse programs.

An Easy-fitness Week

So, what exactly will your easy-fitness life look like? Obviously, everyone has a different schedule at work and at home, and not everyone has plenty of free time to devote to workouts. Every person will also have different preferences when it comes to what type of exercise to do. Nevertheless, what follows is a sample easy-fitness week that will show you how a few 10-minute bursts of activity, coupled with scheduled workouts, can make a previously sedentary life become fitness oriented.

Monday

6:00 A.M.	12:00 P.M.	7:30 P.M.
10-minute abs routine	Walk around block at work	40-minute yoga DVD

Tuesday

6:00 A.M.	12:00 P.M.	7:30 P.M.
10-minute legs-with-weights routine	Walk around block at work	Clean house for one hour; listen to new CD and dance to three songs.

Wednesday

6:00 A.M.	12:00 P.M.	7:30 P.M.
10-minute arms-with-weights routine	Walk around block at work	40-minute yoga DVD

Thursday

6:00 A.M.	12:00 P.M.	7:30 P.M.
10-minute back-and-shoulders-with-weights routine	Walk around block at work	Do laundry; listen to favorite old CD and dance to three songs.

Friday		
6:00 A.M.	12:00 P.M.	7:30 P.M.
10-minute butt-with-weights routine	Walk around block at work	40-minute yoga DVD

After a regimented week, you can take it a little easier on the weekend. For example, on Saturday you might go bowling with friends, and play pool. On Sunday, you could take a 1-hour spinning class. The important thing is that you keep moving, and avoid sitting on the couch all weekend.

Your Nonactive Life

People talk on the phone for hours, they shop, they watch TV—they do a million things without thinking about the time they take. And while these activities often end up taking precedence over exercise, they really shouldn't. Did you know that the average American adult watches TV for around four hours every day? Additionally, TV watching burns fewer calories than any other activity, including sleeping. Is that really how you want to be spending your time?

These things we do—watching TV, playing games on the computer, talking on the phone, and going shopping—are habits, mostly habits we fall into without thinking about it. Few of us plan to spend five hours watching TV, few of us plan to surf the Web during our entire lunch hour, and few us want to look back on our lives and realize we spent so much of it at the mall.

What Stops Activity

The thing is, it's actually pretty tough to become more active—the stores where we shop for food are no longer along one block, but are a car ride away. The schools we go to and that our kids go to aren't a walk away but are instead, yes, you've got it, a car ride away. It seems that most of the things we do these days require a car.

And it's not just about distance; it's also about time. We rush around, rushing requires moving quickly, and, well, cars go faster than our feet. In our world, you can't easily replace driving with walking. In other words, because your busy lifestyle can often encourage you to be sedentary, you need to acknowledge that even mere 10-minute bursts of activity may need to be scheduled into your life.

Take 10 Minutes

You're at the doctor's office and automatically press the button on the elevator. You're at your son's soccer game and sit on a lawn chair while he runs up and down the field. You're watching a *Friends* repeat at 7:00 P.M. At 7:30 P.M., nothing's on that you like, so you flip channels for a half-hour until another favorite program comes on. You see the problem, right? These are all times when you could be moving, rather than not moving. The solution: short bursts of activity will not only keep your metabolism burning, but they also will improve your mood and regulate your hormones.

To incorporate 10 minutes of moderate activity into your life three times a day (or even 20-minute and 10-minute bursts, or one 30-minute burst of activity) you need to notice when you are idle and bored. It's unlikely that you can walk while you're in a meeting or while you're feeding your children, but you can walk when you're waiting, watching, or not really doing something.

Making Your Workouts Count

Effective, heart-pumping, calorie-burning workouts are part of your workout goals. Workouts count when they overload or challenge your body. So you'll need to learn how to make your workouts challenging enough to create changes in your body. One of the best ways to do this is with intervals.

Intervals involve a repeated series of intense exercise workouts interspersed with more moderate exercise periods. Intervals are commonly used to make gains in endurance, strength, speed, or some combination of those, and are used to improve both aerobic and anaerobic performance and conditioning. They are so effective they are like hitting a fast-forward button of progress, as long as they are not overdone. Interval workouts train your body to work more efficiently by using short periods of high-intensity exercise to challenge your typical workout program. Intervals are fun because of their variety and intensity, and your feelings of satisfaction after completing them. Plus, when you use your heart-rate monitor, you can watch your different heart-rate responses.

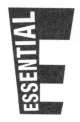

Adapt your exercise time to work with your frequency and intensity. For instance, if you normally exercise five times per week but have a hectic week approaching that allows for only three times per week, you can adjust your exercise time for longer periods to compensate for the lower frequency. Also, if you want to exercise at a higher intensity level than normal, you should shorten your time of exercise accordingly.

Designing Your Own Interval Session

You can design interval sessions for any activity. Here are some key points to consider when planning your interval training session.

- Always include a thorough warm-up.
- Remember that intervals are for limited periods of time, and are not to be practiced for the entire portion of an exercise session.
- Interval sessions should not exceed two times per week.
- The benefits of interval training can be achieved by exercising at intensity levels that are higher aerobic levels, or by crossing the threshold into anaerobic levels.
- To interval train, adjust your exercise session either by increasing the exercise intensity or length of the intense work interval, decreasing the length of the rest and recovery phase, or increasing the number of intervals per session.

When you return to exercise or perform work at the previous aerobic levels, it will feel easier. This is because your cardiovascular system, through the overload principle, has become more efficient. You are now able to do more with less effort. This is a good sign. It means that you are getting more fit and are in better condition.

Tips for Beginners

When the subject is exercise, more is *not* always better. You may not remember this, but before you learned to walk, you had to crawl. Well, the same is true for your fitness. If you want to be successful with your fitness program and want to feel good both during and after exercise, you will need to start in small increments of time and effort, and then increase gradually. This is where many people set themselves up to fail. They expect their bodies to perform activity at levels that are neither realistic nor recommended. Afterward they feel bad, and then wrongly insist that it's the exercise itself that makes them feel worse.

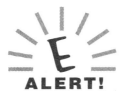
ALERT!

Warm-ups and cooldowns are important, and it is up to you to make sure you incorporate them into your exercise time. A warm-up should last 5 to 10 minutes and get you feeling ready to work. To cool down, reduce the intensity level of exercise gradually, over about 5 minutes.

It is particularly important to start slowly if you have not exercised recently. When you begin an exercise program, you should be gentle with your body. If you start slowly, your body will respond favorably, and you will reinforce the positive effects of your new exercise program. To set yourself up for success, start with small increments of time at low intensity levels until your body has had time to adjust to the new activity.

Activewear

You want to stick with your exercise program, but you don't want your exercise clothing sticking to you! The wrong kind of clothing can cause imprints, chafing, and blisters. Some people mock fashion for exercise (they must be nonexercisers!), but authentic exercise clothing that is designed for function will help you stay with your program.

Does the thought of riding a stationary bike in tight-fitting blue jeans send a chill up your spine? Or how do you like it when your shorts or shirt have chafed your skin? How confident do you feel when you wear worn-out, torn, and faded garments? Does such clothing make you feel more outgoing and friendly, or does it make you want to avoid contact with others? Wearing comfortable, functional, colorful clothing during exercise can greatly enhance your comfort and enjoyment. If you want to elevate your mood while you exercise, wear exercise clothing that feels good, and that you feel good about.

Sports Bras

Unlike the male support garments that have been around a long time, sports bras were first introduced in the late 1970s, but didn't become widely accepted (and even worn without a shirt over them) until the 1980s, as the running boom hit. One of the originals, named the Jogbra, has become for many people the categorical description. Now more universally known as the sports bra, this supportive garment has had a revolutionary impact on women's health and independence. It liberated big-breasted women, who were previously inactive; today, large-breasted women have numerous options for exercising in comfort.

There are three types of sports bras: compression, encapsulation, and combination. The compression style uses fabric pressure to squeeze or press the breasts inward toward the chest, which limits movement. Small- to medium-breasted women favor this style. The encapsulation style limits movement by surrounding and supporting the breasts with reinforced seams or wire, and it is a favorite of large-breasted women. The combination compression-encapsulation sports bra uses both principles.

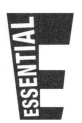

If your local sporting goods or running stores do not have what you need, two women's apparel catalogs with great selections of sports bras are Title Nine Sports and Athleta (see Appendix A for contact information). Brands include Adidas, Champion, Hind, Moving Comfort, Nike, and Reebok. Sports bras cost from $28 to $60.

There are many style and material options for sports bras, and women are all the healthier and happier for them. Comfort should ultimately dictate a woman's choice. The options include underwire, wireless, rear clasp, front clasp, no clasp, front zipper, cross-over the head, cross-in-the-back, cross-in-the-front, halter style, nursing compatible, prosthetic compatible, heart-rate monitor encapsulable, high impact, and low impact. Fabrics include Lycra, Coolmax, Supplex, polyester/Lycra, Drylete, cotton, spandex, and mesh.

Yoga Pants and Tops

Workout pants used to be either restrictively tight, with lots of Lycra, or sweatpants—neither of which is attractive on the majority of people, male or female. Within the past five years, however, the popularity of yoga has liberated the workout pant and given us yoga pants. Yoga pants are shapely but not skin tight, and usually have nice patterns and a variety of lengths. Even though they are called yoga pants, you can use them for any activity, even spinning. Yoga tops are also often comfortable for women because they stretch but aren't skin tight.

Not Just Cotton

Exercise and 100 percent cotton garments have outgrown each other as optimum partners. Why? Because 100 percent cotton items become wet and stay wet, which can cause chafing, odor, and chills. New fabrics are used in every form of exercise clothing on the market, including shirts, tops, undershirts, vests, jackets, arm warmers, hats, earmuffs, headbands, sports bras, shorts, tights, leg warmers, sweats, compression shorts, socks, swimsuits, and wetsuits. Wearing 100 percent cotton exercise clothing is the equivalent of using rotary-dial telephones. You can still use them, but your options are severely limited. Older fabrics are not as efficient, productive, or comfortable as the newer ones.

New fabrics speed up the evaporation of perspiration, which keeps you dry, temperature regulated, and comfortable. This moisture-wicking action also makes you less "nose-able," that is, less noticeable in an odoriferous way. The moisture-releasing properties make laundering these garments easier because they dry quickly. This can be a big plus when you only have a few athletic garments, are traveling, or need to wash and wear the same clothes again the very next day. So select newer fabrics for your exercise clothes, and experience their many comforts and conveniences.

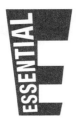

The blended, engineered fabrics to look for in your exercise clothing are Coolmax, Drylete, Lycra, polypropylene, polyester, spandex, Supplex, cotton blends, wool, and wool blends. These work to move moisture away from the body, allowing you to stay dry and fresh, and avoid uncomfortable chafing and blisters.

Socks

Some people tend to take socks for granted. But it only takes one blister to bring your feet to your attention. Socks are meant to support your body, reduce friction, regulate foot temperature, and promote comfort and circulation. The fit of your socks can make a tremendous difference in your exercise comfort. Your socks should not constrict your skin or make a deep imprint on it, especially at the ankles or calves. Socks should not bunch up inside your shoes or slide off your feet, and you should be able to move your feet and wiggle your toes comfortably.

Again, 100 percent cotton, once recommended, is no longer the winner. Socks made from Coolmax, Supplex, Kevlar, acrylic, merino wool, wool blends, combed cotton, nylon, or cotton blends help keep moisture, blistering, and bunching to a minimum, all of which leads to greater overall comfort. A high-performance sock label reads like the chemistry panel for a scientific experiment, but these are highly functional, comfortable socks designed for long-term wear and endurance athletics.

Shoes

Shoes support your body weight, so you definitely want the right shoe for your specific activity. Some simple ailments of the ankles, hips, and knees are easily avoided by wearing the appropriate shoe. For fitness activities whose foot movements are largely up and down and compression related, such as standing or pedaling, an average running shoe will provide excellent support. For activities whose movements are predominantly lateral, such as aerobics or racket sports, either a sport-specific shoe (a tennis shoe for tennis) or a cross-trainer is appropriate. Go to a shoe store specializing in sports shoes to get the right advice about which shoe to buy, as the salespeople in those stores are educated about what the proper fit should be and how to match activities to shoes.

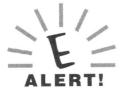

ALERT!

Don't be fooled! Just because it looks like a sneaker doesn't mean it is meant for exercise. Flat rubber-soled shoes without support are not necessarily what you need for walks. If you have any doubts, head to a fitness store and ask for advice from their salespeople.

When you go to buy new shoes, wear the socks you plan to wear with the shoes, and go to the shoe store later in the day, as your feet will be slightly larger than they are in the morning. Try on a number of different brands, as they are all sized slightly differently. Some brands, such as New Balance, are made slightly wider than others. If you plan to take part in a few activities, don't hesitate to buy appropriate shoes for each one, although cross-trainers will work for most sports, except perhaps tennis or other sports on specialty courts and surfaces.

Putting It All Together

Some moms bake homemade cookies, and some moms order take-out. Some moms are triathletes, and some moms can't find 10 minutes for themselves. Becoming a fit and active person doesn't mean that you need to go to the gym or become a runner. The only thing it means is that you need to figure out how you and your life can be active in a way that works for you and makes you happy.

Fit people who enjoy exercise usually have a number of activities and ways to exercise so they can get their fix in. But very often, before people get started, they are concerned about their limitations, such as time and money.

The following are some common exercise concerns and issues, and their solutions.

Issue	Solution
Don't have enough time?	Work out at home, do 10-minute bursts of exercise.
Afraid to be seen in shorts?	Do yoga, dance (at night, in skirts), work out at home.
Work long, odd hours?	Get in 10-minute bursts, exercise when you wake up, join a 24-hour gym.
Travel a lot?	Use body weight/resistance bands; learn yoga, Pilates.
Need time for yourself?	Do yoga, learn Pilates, run, swim.
Want to socialize?	Take group exercise classes, compete in races.
Competitive?	Learn martial arts, compete in races.
Want to learn a skill?	Take classes in horseback riding, rowing, kayaking, rock climbing, gymnastics, and ballet.
Sit down all day?	Walk, run, dance, do yoga, learn Pilates, swim, take ballet, have fun with most sports.
Easily bored?	Learn a new sport or ballet, then cross-train.
Broke?	Walk, run, dance, go to parks, rent exercise DVDs from the library.

Very often, when people set goals, they focus on the end result, such as "I want to lose ten pounds" or "I want to wear size eight jeans." These statements aren't helpful, though, because they don't include an action, or a way to actually reach the goal. How are you going to lose the ten pounds or wear smaller jeans? You need a detailed plan to reach a goal. So, let's first focus on creating an active intention, which is much more likely to lead to success.

For example, you could create an intention of walking 20 minutes every day when you wake up. Or you could set the intention to use one segment of a DVD that has collections of 10-minute workouts on it. More than anything else, intentions are doable; they aren't wishful thinking. The following is a list of sample active intentions you can use as a model for your own:

- Take two step aerobics classes this week.
- Garden on Sunday morning.
- Walk after dinner three nights this week.
- Take a bike ride on Saturday.
- Go dancing Friday night.

The good news is that the ultimate result of an active intention is often something you want, such as losing weight or wearing smaller jeans. If you walk every day, you'll probably lose weight if you begin to strength train; you'll fit into smaller jeans, and even more important, if you become more active, you'll be fitter.

Now that you know about the overload principle, FITT, and some of what your fitness requirements will be to stay healthy and lose weight, write down some active intentions that will allow you to see immediate results. One can be fun, like buying workout pants. One can be easy, like making sure you walk ten minutes on your lunch hour; and one can be challenging, like taking a new class or going for a hike this Saturday.

Once you achieve those first goals, grab a notebook and jot down three more active intentions. Your intentions should be short term, covering from tomorrow through the week. This way, you'll be able to ensure that you can reach them. And don't forget to reward yourself! Then, the next week, write three new active intentions. You'll find that, over time, your intentions will become more intense and challenging as you see how easy it is to reach your goals this way.

Chapter 3
Walking

More people walk for exercise than do any other activity. And that's great, because as activities go, walking is safe, effective, easy, and fun. But that doesn't mean everyone walks properly or understands how to make their walks into effective workouts. The only way walking will help your heart and your waistline is when it's done with intention and intensity. This chapter will serve as your introduction to the world of walking, and teach you how to take your walking to the next level.

Walking: Low-impact Aerobics

When you walk, one foot is always in contact with the ground, which makes it a low-impact aerobic activity. Walking will not forcibly jar your skeletal system, but because it is a weight-bearing activity, it stimulates bone growth and density. This, in turn, helps prevent osteoporosis. You can walk nearly anywhere: in the city, in the country, in a neighborhood, in a shopping mall, or for transportation.

Walking builds muscular strength and endurance in your legs, arms (if swung properly), and the muscles of the back and abdomen that keep your trunk erect. It also improves coordination and balance. Besides being easy, walking has a meditative quality that calms the mind and fights depression and anxiety, and you can do it alone or with another person or in a group.

Walking Shoes

Despite what you may have heard, not just any old shoes are suitable for walking. You need shoes that provide support in all the right places. Good walking shoes help support and protect your spine, hips, knees, ankles, and feet. One unnecessary trip to the doctor is more expensive than what it costs for a decent pair of walking shoes, so do not hesitate to buy them. Buy shoes that are truly meant for walking. Avoid aerobic or court shoes because they do not provide the type of support needed for walking. If you are a combination walker and jogger, you may choose to get running shoes instead. But if you are exclusively a walker, again, get a pair of walking shoes. Walking shoes offer a bit more flexibility, which you need because when you walk, you flex your feet and push off with your toes more than when you run.

Because you land on your heels, you need a stable shoe that has a heel counter, the cuplike device in the heel of the shoe that helps to secure your foot and keep it from moving around. Although it's good to incorporate walking into your daily routines and errands, it is best not to walk as rigorously or for as long a period of time in your dress or street shoes as you would when walking strictly for exercise. Your feet will pay the price with pain, blisters, or both.

Proper Walking Posture

To walk properly, imagine a cord coming out of the center and top of your head that gently pulls you up straight. One of the most common errors walkers make is leaning forward rather than standing erect. Keep your hips directly under your upper body. You don't want to be stiff, but you should avoid bending at your hips or hunching your shoulders. Another common error is walking with the head down, looking at the ground immediately in front of the feet. Keep your head up and look several feet *ahead* of where your feet are landing.

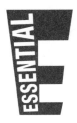

Aside from the need for walking shoes to help reduce the chance of injury or pain, walking is cheap and easy. If you walk regularly and use good shoes, walking can build abdominal strength and leg strength. It has little or no learning curve, and you can improve your skills and effectiveness over time.

When you walk, your arms should be relaxed (taking deep breaths helps) and balanced so that the actions of both arms are the same. Swing your arms counter to your legs—in other words, move your right arm when you are moving your left leg, and move your left arm when you are moving your right leg. Keep your arms bent to about a 90-degree angle, and hold them close to your body rather than having them wing out. Swinging your arms will also help you to elevate your heart rate. While your arms should swing, your hands shouldn't go across the midline of the body or above the level of your chest. Hold your hands with the thumbs up, and with a loose fist.

How to Get Started

If you are just beginning a walking program, go out and walk for a short period of time, maybe 10 minutes. Check in with your body the next day, and if all systems are go, then repeat the 10-minute walking period. Gradually increase the time of your walk, perhaps in 5-minute increments over a period of days, or weeks if necessary. If you are feeling pretty good and pain free, you can walk on consecutive days, but if pain or soreness is a problem, then either select a different activity or rest completely for a day or so.

Continue to check in with your body for any soreness, aches, or pains. Soreness is natural when you are just getting started; pain is not. When the soreness is light, you can continue to increase walking time. Over time, you can build up to 30 minutes or even an hour of walking and can increase from walking every other day to nearly every day.

Don't Carry Weights

Carrying weights in your hands while walking (heavy hands) was conceptually a good idea for helping to elevate the heart rate and build muscular strength. However, the reality is that it has caused many people joint problems in the elbows, wrists, and shoulders. If you want to elevate your heart rate, walk faster, walk on a course with some hills, or walk with a weighted backpack. If you want to strengthen your upper body, see Chapter 8 to learn how to strength train. But mixing weights with walking is not the way to go.

Pace Yourself

Pace refers to the number of minutes it takes to complete each mile; *miles per hour* refers to the number of miles you would cover at that pace in an hour. Sometimes you will want to know your pace, and sometimes the miles per hour. Use these steps to convert them back and forth as needed.

To convert pace to miles per hour:
1. First, convert your pace (in seconds or minutes) to a decimal (in minutes). For example, 45 seconds = .75 minute; 30 seconds = .50 minute; 15 seconds = .25 minute; 10 seconds = .166 minute; 13 ½ minutes per mile = 13.5.
2. Next, divide the number 60 by the pace (as a decimal) to get the miles per hour. For example: 60 ÷ 13.5 = 4.44 miles per hour. This tells you that at a 13 ½-minute pace, you would cover 4.44 miles in an hour.

To convert miles per hour to pace:

Divide the number 60 by the miles per hour (as a decimal) to determine the pace as a decimal. For example: 60 ÷ 4.44 mph = 13.51 minute pace. This tells you that walking at a speed of 4.44 mph, it takes you 13 ½ minutes to cover each mile.

As you progress to longer and more intense walks, consider using a heart-rate monitor to gauge your intensity level and to motivate you to move at a good clip, but not to overdo it. Or set some goals for time, speed, and distance and occasionally test yourself to see your progress. Check your heart rate during exercise and your recovery heart rate. When you see those numbers improving, then it is time to overload yourself to make even further improvements.

You can also vary your pace by speeding up for short intervals of time or distance. Treat yourself to the fun experience of signing up for a walking or jogging event such as a 5k (1 kilometer = .625 of a mile) or 10k. Having such a goal will motivate you, and participating will definitely increase how much you enjoy your walking program, and the seriousness with which you view it.

10,000 Steps a Day

Many people are now trying to ensure they take at least 10,000 steps per day, which has been shown to be a marker of good health. If you walk about 3.5 miles per hour, then you probably take somewhere between 5,000 and 7,000 steps in one hour, depending on your height (and, therefore, your stride length). You can walk that number of steps during a one-hour show on TV just by marching in front of your TV. You'll burn about 150 to 250 calories during that hour. That may not sound like a lot, but if you're just watching TV without moving, you'll only burn about 40 to 60 calories, and not get any boost to your metabolism during that time. Do that for one hour a day for a year, and you'll burn off about 9 pounds!

Of course, you can also buy a step counter, or pedometer, which you can hook onto your pants (at the waistband) or your shoes. These little doodads, which have become so popular that McDonald's was giving them away for a while, are supposed to be an easy way to help you make sure you're getting your 10,000 steps in. The problem is that these machines are often inaccurate, so they either overcount or undercount your steps. Nevertheless, they aren't expensive and they do work for some people, so you might try one out. Take 100 steps (count), and then see how close the piece of equipment is. If it's pretty close (maybe 95 to 105 steps) then use it. If not, try to make estimates yourself.

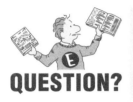

QUESTION?

Where can I get a pedometer, and how much do they generally cost?
You can buy a pedometer at pretty much any retail sports shop, or online. There are seemingly countless online retailers that sell pedometers; for example, visit *www.everythingfitness.com* and *www.amazon .com*. Pedometers often cost somewhere between $5 and $30, depending on their features. Some even include an FM radio.

Long Walks Versus Short Bursts

If 30 minutes of brisk walking burns about 75 calories and strengthens your abs, heart, and leg muscles, what does 10 minutes of walking plus 10 minutes of walking plus 10 minutes of walking do? The very same thing, of course. The only difference between getting your walking done in short bursts versus long ones is that you won't build cardiovascular and muscular endurance with short bursts of walking (or any other exercise, for that matter). But if you are really time pressed, don't worry. Just make your walks 10 minutes. The benefits aren't exactly the same, but they are good enough. And walking is better than doing nothing, even if it's just for 10 minutes.

Eventually, you'll want to work your way up to longer walks, but more than that, you'll want to find a variety of ways to make your walks more intense in terms of calorie burning and heart conditioning. Adding an incline, such as with hill climbing, stair climbing, and hiking, can help you achieve this.

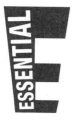

Short walks contribute to overall health, but they do not constitute fitness workouts. However, short walks are a great addition to an exercise program for mood elevation and for keeping your metabolism rolling along throughout the day. For example, try taking short walks to split up your workday. Take a quick 10-minute walk in the midmorning, a 15-minute walk at lunchtime, and another 10-minute walk in the midafternoon. You'll get a burst of energy, and will probably notice an increase in your productivity.

Adding an Incline

Adding an incline (in other words, simulating walking uphill) to your walks will help you in two ways. First, it gets your heart pumping, increasing the intensity level of your workout without increasing the impact on your joints. Second, climbing works your butt and leg muscles like nothing else, sculpting your glutes and hamstrings until they are sleek and lean.

Stair Climbing

Stair climbing is a fun, easy way to introduce some incline into your walking routine. One of the best ways to use stair climbing is by adding it during a 10-minute break in your day. You'll burn a lot of calories (in 10 minutes, anyway) and keep your heart pumping long after you stop going up the stairs (going down is good, too, by the way). Many office buildings have stairs, of course, and you can easily design a route that will allow you to walk through the building without anyone thinking you are just wasting time. If you need to make a copy, for example, take the scenic route to get to the copier, and then take a different route back to your desk. No one will be the wiser, and your body will thank you.

Hiking

Rest assured, hiking doesn't necessarily refer to backpacking, i.e., carrying a heavy pack on your back, and walking for miles up into the mountains.

For your purposes, all hiking means is heading to the mountains or even walking on a flat path while you're wearing trail shoes.

Trail shoes look like a combination of sneakers and mountain boots. They are lighter than boots, but have treads that allow you to walk on rocks and dirt. They are an absolute necessity for hiking—sneakers just won't do the job. Most good sneaker companies make trail shoes, too, and most good shoe stores (not department stores, but sporting goods stores) have many choices. Try them on with appropriate socks, i.e., ones with cushioning that will allow your foot to breathe. And remember that after a few hours of hiking, your feet will swell a bit, so you need your trail shoes to be roomy.

The Trusty Treadmill

Once you get used to the feeling of the ground moving beneath your feet, you can truly appreciate walking and running on a treadmill. The treadmill is obedient and will keep the speed and level of incline steady. Intensity is determined by the speed and incline settings. You can either control the settings yourself through the manual mode or experiment with the pre-programmed workouts. Many home models will allow you to program your own workouts and keep them in memory so you can repeat them.

Here's another bonus about using a treadmill: You can choose to run or to walk. If you are a runner who wants to walk on the treadmill but have difficulty elevating your heart rate, walk your fingers over to the inclination control and press "up." Your heart rate will go up quickly in response to even slight incline changes such as 1 to 2 percent. Do not focus so much on your heart rate that you forget about your muscles, which may not be used to a higher inclination. Increase the incline gradually and give your muscles time to adjust. The muscles used while walking on a high incline are different from those used when running.

If the increase in the incline doesn't agree with your hips, knees, or ankles, but you still want to elevate your heart rate while walking, wear a backpack and put some light weight in it. You can use a telephone book or weight plates. but use small weights such as 1 to 5 pounds. Just carrying that seemingly small amount will elevate your heart rate. It will also give you an appreciation for what it would feel like if you weighed that much more and had to carry it around with you all the time.

The treadmill makes for an efficient workout because it eliminates the distractions that outdoor exercise can pose (traffic, road debris, etc.) and allows you to maintain intensity. A good treadmill has a shock-absorbing pad built into the platform that makes the force absorbed by the body gentler than what your body would absorb from concrete or asphalt pavement outdoors. You should avoid holding the handrails continuously during exercise; use them mostly to steady yourself or regain your balance.

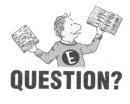

QUESTION?

Is it worth it to use the fat-burning setting on my treadmill?
No. By using this setting, you will exercise at a lower intensity. Even though you burn higher percentages of fat, rather than glucose (sugar), when you exercise at a lower intensity, the bottom line is that the harder you work out, the more calories you burn, and the more calories you burn, the more fat you burn overall.

Before using a treadmill, you must learn how to control it. After all, it's a self-propelled machine that can get ahead of you if you're not prepared. Follow these guidelines to ensure your safety:

- Know where the stop button or the emergency pull cord is located.
- Practice grabbing the handrail and straddling both feet so that they rest on the nonmoving side panels. Then stop the machine or turn the intensity down before you put your feet on the central part of the treadmill again.
- Do not look directly down at your feet. Stay focused and avoid turning your body, even if your kids are calling you.
- A moving treadmill can be dangerous to curious children, pets, and so on. Keep them away from it, and keep the operating key out of reach when the machine is not in use.

- Position the back of the treadmill away from a wall so that even if you slip on the treadmill, you don't have to worry about hitting anything solid.

Begin each treadmill session by walking slowly for 5 minutes. Then gradually increase the speed and inclination to your desired levels. Most treadmills have display settings—for your speed, inclination, the distance covered, and approximate calories burned—that will entertain you while you walk or run. You can use the information to challenge yourself by keeping track of your progress. Pace is another motivating unit of measure.

The Elliptical Trainer: A New Walking Alternative

If you love walking but want to kick up your workouts a notch without sacrificing your joints and without having to bounce, try an elliptical trainer. Elliptical trainers provide an effective cardiovascular workout, work all the major muscle groups in the leg, and do so with low impact upon your joints. They can be programmed to move in forward or backward motions. The backward motion emphasizes the gluteal muscles (buttocks), but since the legs aren't meant to move in that direction at a fast pace, stick with a forward motion, as if you're walking or running.

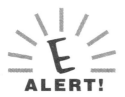

Leaning on the handles or using moving arm poles on the elliptical trainer won't increase your calorie burning or workout intensity. In fact, leaning on the machine will actually decrease the intensity of your workout. Let go of the handles and, if you can, move as if you're walking or running (i.e., swing your arms naturally).

There are two important things to know about elliptical trainers. First, you can adapt almost any walking and running program to these machines. While you can't exactly match a treadmill's speed in miles per hour to the elliptical trainer's pace measurements (done in steps), you can incorporate intervals and resistance on the elliptical trainer. Also, most people do about 130 steps per minute on an elliptical trainer, so you can push yourself to higher speeds—150 or 160 steps per minute—that are the equivalent of walking faster.

Jogging and Running

The difference between jogging and running is mainly intensity. Jogging is a slower, less intense version of running. Running is moving with quick steps on alternate feet, and never having both feet on the ground at the same time. Running is one of the most popular aerobic activities. Even short jogs can be helpful in increasing your metabolism and in burning more calories than you would on a walk. Adding five or six 30-second jogs to your walk can be extremely beneficial to your overall speed and intensity, too.

As compared to most aerobic activities, running uses more liters of oxygen minute for minute. And since the body expends 5 calories for every liter of oxygen processed, running is an efficient way to burn calories and manage body fat and weight. Running is also an effective means of producing endorphins—those feel-good hormones—so much so that the term *runner's high* is often used to describe the endorphin effect.

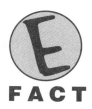

FACT

Running does not require many skills, but technique is important. Because of the increased gravitational force absorbed by the body, technique is even more important than in walking. When you run, keep your head up and your eyes focused a little ahead of you rather than directly in front of you. Keep your abs gently contracted so that you are holding your torso tall, and keep your shoulders relaxed and away from your ears. Be sure your knees are bent when your feet land.

Running is a high-impact aerobic activity that has both good and bad effects on the body. It is good because it stimulates bone growth and density, but at the same time, running jars the skeletal system. You can also run nearly anywhere and cover a lot of turf in a short amount of time. You can conveniently run when you are traveling. It is a great way to explore new areas, as long as you have a good enough sense of direction to get you back to where you started. Running builds muscular strength and endurance of the entire body, especially the hips, legs, and feet. These are only some of the reasons why running is such a preferred aerobic activity. Talk to runners, and they will share with you how they love running and what it does for their psyches.

But unfortunately, if you run too far or too frequently, you increase the possibility of musculoskeletal injuries or overuse syndromes. Common injuries to the knees, hips, and Achilles tendons are often the result of too much running. Listen to your own body and don't compare what is too much for you to what is too much for someone else. If you plan to run for your main aerobic exercise activity, make sure you stretch after your run and, if it feels good to you, stretch after the first few minutes of running, too. It can also be helpful to alternate other aerobic activities with running and to plan for rest days.

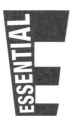

Water bottles make drinking while moving easy. But what about when you don't have one handy? Take the lead from experienced runners who have mastered the art of drinking out of paper cups on the fly. Squeeze the top of the paper cup to form a "V" and pour directly into your mouth.

If you run on a trail, let someone know where you are going, and when you plan to leave and expect to return. For safety reasons, women should consider finding companions to accompany them when running in unpopulated areas. Dogs and human companions can be fun additions to running, and they provide security.

Chapter 4

Ten Effective Walking Programs

Now that you know the basics of walking for fitness, it's time to focus on the next step: walking programs. You can do a different program every day, or find one or two you like and alternate them. It's best to not do the same walk every day, though, because your body gets used to workouts and needs to be challenged by new routines to continue seeing results. These programs include things like stretching, weights, lunges, and more.

30-minute Intervals

Intervals are workouts that include alternating segments of high- and moderate-intensity exercise. Intervals are incredibly effective, and anyone can do them because the intense segments only have to be harder than your typical workout, and not as hard as, say, what a professional athlete might do. For example, if you are someone who typically walks at a snail's pace, then upping your intensity could mean walking at a turtle pace. The important thing is that you're challenging yourself to work harder than you typically work. These intervals give you a way to increase your overall walking pace, while, at the same time, increasing your caloric burn and cardiovascular strengthening during one workout.

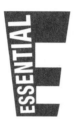

To find out how fast you're walking, count your steps (both feet) for 20 seconds (use the second hand on a watch, or a stopwatch). If you count 40, you're walking about 3 mph (which is good for your health, but not your fitness). If you're up to 45, you're walking 3.5 to 4 mph, which will lead to weight loss. Get up to 50, and you're walking to improve your heart.

Here's another great thing about intervals—they don't have to last long to be effective. Even 30 seconds at a faster-than-normal pace will do your heart and your calorie burning goals a whole lot of good. Of course, the longer and harder your exercise, the more effective the workout is, but, once again, if you're not in terrific shape, even a 30-second interval can improve your heart health, up your fitness level, and increase your caloric burn exponentially.

There's one more great thing about interval workouts: You can increase your intensity in a variety of ways. For example, to make segments of your walk more intense, you can jog, climb a hill, add a weighted vest, or walk faster.

Walking with a Weighted Vest

Backpacks often aren't attractive. Their weight is often unevenly distributed. And it's difficult to be sure exactly how much weight you are carrying. With a weighted vest you can control exactly how much you are carrying, which will easily allow you to increase that weight when you're ready.

Wearing a weighted vest increases the intensity of your workout, so you don't need to use intervals. And because of the higher intensity, the walks can be shorter than other walks if your focus is on strengthening your heart.

This program uses the Rating of Perceived Exertion (RPE) to gauge workout intensity. Revisit Chapter 1 for details of RPE. At the end of each session, be sure to remove the vest and stretch.

Week One (Do the following four times a week):

Vest	Put 5 pounds in vest.
Warm-up	Walk slowly for 5 minutes, gradually getting up to a moderate speed.
Workout	Walk for 20 minutes on a flat surface, staying at a speed that keeps your RPE at 6 or above.
Cooldown	Move from a moderate speed to a slow speed.

Week Two (Do the following four times a week):

Vest	Put 10 pounds in vest.
Warm-up	Walk slowly for 5 minutes, gradually getting up to a moderate speed.
Workout	Walk for 20 minutes on a flat surface, staying at a speed that keeps your RPE between 6 and 7.
Cooldown	Move from a moderate speed to a slow speed.

Week Three (Do the following four times a week):

Vest	Put 10 pounds in vest.
Warm-up	Walk slowly for 5 minutes, moving up to a moderate speed.

Workout	Find a place to walk with hills or stairs. Walk for 5 minutes on a flat surface, staying at an RPE of 5 to 6. After 5 minutes, climb a hill or climb the stairs for 2 minutes. Go back to the flat surface for 5 minutes. Do this four times.
Cooldown	For the next 5 minutes, move from a moderate speed to a slow speed.

Week Four (Do the following four times a week):

Vest	Put 10 pounds in vest.
Warm-up	Walk slowly for 5 minutes, gradually getting up to a moderate speed.
Workout	Find a place with hills or stairs. Walk for 4 minutes on a flat surface, staying at a speed that keeps your RPE between 5 and 6. Go to the hill or stairs and walk up them for 4 minutes. Go back to the flat surface. Do this four times.
Cooldown	For the next 5 minutes, move from a moderate speed to a slow speed.

Jogging a 5k

Over the last few years, an amazing thing has happened to the world of 5ks (and other races, even marathons). Walkers have begun taking part in races that used to be reserved for runners, and, even more interesting perhaps, runners have begun incorporating walking into their races to make their bodies less prone to injury and to actually improve their race times! Paradoxically, the walking intervals allow the runners to maintain an overall faster speed because their bodies aren't being stressed so much throughout the race.

In all ways except two this workout is an interval program. The differences are that you are working toward a goal, and that you are thinking in terms of miles, not minutes for your intervals.

The following is a seven-week program. Even if you don't have a regular walking schedule now, following this program will still enable you to take part in a race very soon.

Week	Mon	Tue	Wed	Thu	Fri	Sat	Sun
1	Rest or jog/run	1.5 mile run	Rest or jog/run	1.5 mile run	Rest	1.5 mile run	60 min walk
2	Rest or jog/run	1.75 mile run	Rest or jog/run	1.5 mile run	Rest	1.75 mile run	60 min walk
3	Rest or jog/run	2 mile run	Rest or jog/run	1.5 mile run	Rest	2 mile run	60 min walk
4	Rest or jog/run	2.25 mile run	Rest or jog/run	1.5 mile run	Rest	2.25 mile run	60 min walk
5	Rest or jog/run	2.5 mile run	Rest or jog/run	2 mile run	Rest	2.5 mile run	60 min walk
6	Rest or jog/run	2.75 mile run	Rest or jog/run	2 mile run	Rest	2.75 mile run	60 min walk
7	Rest or jog/run	3 mile run	Rest or jog/run	2 mile run	Rest	1 mile run	Race

Fartlek Walk

Fartlek means "fast play" in Swedish. It's possibly the easiest way to do an interval workout, which makes it the most fun, and yet it's as effective as any other workout. During a Fartlek workout, you'll do bursts of fast walking (or running, if you're so inclined) using landmarks as your interval guides. So, for example, let's say you're walking around your neighborhood. You could walk at an easy pace for 5 minutes as your warm-up. Then look ahead for a landmark, such as a telephone pole, tree, mailbox, or corner. Now run or walk fast to that spot. Go back to walking at a moderate pace once you get to your landmark to give yourself time to recover and bring your heart rate down to normal. Then pick another landmark, and jog or walk fast to it. Repeat this three or four times during your 30-minute workout.

Each time you do this workout, your speed during your jogging or fast-walking intervals will increase because your fitness level will improve, and also your speed during your walk intervals will improve, too.

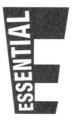

Once your walks are going faster, you can improve them in another way. Instead of just stopping your walk at its usual end, add on another Fartlek interval, which will increase the workout's effectiveness by adding both length and intensity. Of course, you could also increase the length of each Fartlek interval by, say, running past the Coopers' driveway (where you had usually stopped running before) and going all the way down to the Finklesteins.'

The next time you're on a walk, look around for landmarks that would work in a Fartlek program. Then, the next time you walk, go for those intervals. Don't try to be an Olympic-level athlete. Just jog or walk as fast as you can to each landmark. You'll feel the difference in your breathing rate, and most likely just in the way you feel—more energetic, most likely.

Endurance Walk

Endurance means duration or the length of a workout, but an extra-long workout is effective only if the intensity level of the workout is already high enough. In other words, don't think that length is a substitute for…well, anything else. In an endurance workout, you're going to do intervals or walk at a fast pace or climb some hills, and do it for longer than you usually do.

So if you typically walk for 30 minutes, your endurance walk will be for 45 or 60 minutes, and the majority of that time will be spent at a moderate to high intensity. Follow these steps:

1. Warm up by walking at an easy pace.
2. Walk at a moderate (not easy) pace, feeling your body get warmer and warmer as you increase your pace slightly every few minutes over 20 minutes. By the last 5 minutes, you should be sweaty and breathing deeply.
3. Take a 2-minute recovery period, reducing speed just enough to breathe a little easier.

4. Increase your walking speed again and proceed as you did in step 2 for 20 minutes more, now with even greater intensity.
5. Cool down by gradually slowing down your walk.

Treadmill Walk

While there is nothing quite as peaceful and yet energizing as a walk outside, a treadmill walk has a lot to offer someone who wants to improve her fitness level. For one thing, you can consciously and consistently control your workout speed. You can also control the intensity by increasing the ramp, or angle, or incline, at which you are walking. So, for example, if you are trying to walk faster for a longer period of time, when you do that on a treadmill you can keep track of how far you are walking in a certain time period. It's harder to do that on a street.

Follow these steps for a great treadmill program:

1. Warm up by walking at an easy pace.
2. Walk at incline level 4 or 5 for 5 consecutive minutes. Your breathing should be strong and deep.
3. Reduce the incline and walk easily for recovery (catching your breath) for 2 minutes.
4. Walk at a 1 percent incline, starting at a moderate pace but increasing speed and the incline level every minute for 5 minutes. You should be at a quick pace and 5 percent incline, and breathing strenuously, by the end of your 5 minutes.
5. Do 2 minutes of recovery walking by either slowing down, lowering the incline, or both.
6. Repeat step 3, step 4, and step 3 again.
7. Cool down by returning to a slower walk and lowering the incline gradually.

Uphill Hiking

Because walking for a long time can be boring to some people, another endurance option is to do something fun and loose, such as going on an uphill hike. This way, your intensity will be high enough (because you're climbing a hill), and you'll be engaged in the scenery and the climb itself.

There is no one way to do a hike, i.e., there is no program to follow. All you need to do is follow the trail. However, here is some important information about staying safe and making your walk more effective:

- Be sure you are wearing the right shoes or boots. They should have heavy treads so you don't slip on rocks or dirt, be roomy enough so that your feet have the space they need, and be supportive enough so that you won't turn your ankle.
- After you walk for the first few minutes, take some time to stretch. It will loosen you up and keep your risk of injury down during your hike.
- Bring snacks, water, a trail map, a cell phone, tissues, and a couple of plastic bags, at a minimum. Good snacks include peanut butter sandwiches, trail mix, string cheese and crackers, and fruit. Make sure you eat a good breakfast before you leave, too.
- At a minimum, take a few walks during the weeks before your hike so that your body is somewhat used to walking.
- Stop along the way. In other words, don't rush through your hike. Enjoy yourself.
- Stretch or do a little yoga at the end of your hike. It will reduce soreness the next day.

Walk or Run on a Track

One of the most convenient and useful places to walk—and eventually run— is a high-school (or any other type of school) track. Convenient, because most towns have tracks even if they don't have sidewalks. Useful because you'll know exactly how far you're walking, and there are usually bleachers.

Bleachers turn a walk into a workout. First, you can run or even walk up them to burn more calories and tone your butt in a way nothing else can. Second, you can actually do some exercises on them to work your whole body.

Most tracks are a quarter mile long, so you can quantify your walk in a number of ways. You can time how long it takes you to walk that quarter–mile, and try to walk faster and longer each time. Or you can figure out how long you want to walk and just try to do that walk faster each time. Or you can just try to go a longer distance.

But the best thing to do might be a well-rounded 40-minute workout like this:

1. Warm up by walking around the track once.
2. Walk quickly around the track once.
3. Jog as far as you can, then walk around the rest of the track. Do this eight times.
4. Go over to the bleachers. Walk up the steps. Come down quickly.
5. Now walk up the seats of the bleachers (if they are benches). Or, if you can, take the steps two at a time. Come down. Do this four times.
6. Go to the bottom of the steps to do some lunges, pushups, dips, squats, and ab exercises (see the following descriptions).

Lunges

Put your right foot on the bottom bleacher and step back with your left foot. Your right knee should be slightly bent. Bend your left knee into a lunge while your right knee is also bent, but your left knee shouldn't go past your ankle or toes. You can keep your hands by your sides, or bend your elbows and raise your arms up to your shoulders. Do this lunge sixteen times. Then stand on your left leg and bend your right knee, bringing your right foot toward your butt. Hold on to your foot. This will stretch your quadriceps muscle. Do the lunge on the other side (with your left foot on the bleacher) and then stretch your left quadriceps.

Pushups

Put both hands on the bottom bleacher and then step about three feet away, getting into a pushup position. Make sure you are a straight line from your head to your heels. Exhale, bend your elbows, and come down toward the step, keeping your eyes looking forward toward the next step. On an inhale, come up. Try to do this five times, working your way up to sixteen. When you've finished, stretch your arms out to the side, toward your back, while making sure you keep your shoulders pressed away from your ears, to stretch out your chest.

Dips

Sit down on the lowest bench. Put your hands on either side of your hips, and slide your butt off the seat as you stretch your legs straight out in front of you, heels on the ground, toes pointing up. Keep your shoulders away from your ears, and contract your abs. Bend your elbows and lower your torso down toward the ground, keeping your elbows in. Straighten your arms and come up. Try to do this up to sixteen times. You should feel this in your triceps (the backs of your arms) so when you're done, stand up and bring your right arm up and behind your head. Bend your elbow, dropping your forearm behind your head, and put your left hand on your right elbow. Press down a little to stretch your tricep. If this exercise ever gets too easy, you can always do another set of dips.

Squats

Stand a foot or two in front of the bleachers, facing away from them. Keeping your shoulders away from your ears and your abs contracted, bend your knees and squat down, bringing your butt close to—but not touching—the bleacher. This should take two counts. Hold at the bottom for another two counts, then come up, which should take yet another two counts. Do this sixteen times. To stretch, turn around and face the bleachers. Put your hands on the bottom bleacher and, maintaining your balance, put your right foot on your left knee and bend your left knee. You'll feel this stretch in your butt. If this exercise gets too easy, you can do another set (or two).

Knee-ups

Sit on the first bleacher, legs out, hands by your hips, shoulders down, abs contracted. Lean back a bit and pick your feet up off the ground. Keeping your abs tight and your legs together, bend your knees and bring them in toward your chest. Straighten them again. Repeat fifteen times. Do this slowly.

Twists

Sit on the first bleacher, legs out, shoulders down, abs contracted, arms at shoulder height in a circle (fingertips together, elbows apart). Lean your torso back, keeping your abs together. Now, turn to your right and, as you do this, move your right arm to the right and look to the right. Come back to center and repeat to the left. Do this fifteen times on each side. At the end of these two ab moves, stand up, contract your abs a bit, and relax your shoulders. Then reach your arms up, keeping your shoulders down, and lean back, pushing your hips forward a bit. Hold this for 20 to 30 seconds. Come back to the start position, and keeping your arms over your head, tilt your torso to the right. Hold this for 20 to 30 seconds. Repeat to the left.

Treadmill Challenge

This is a walk designed to mimic one with hills or steps. Your incline level will depend on your treadmill. Most treadmills have inclines that range from 1 to 10 and can be increased in increments of 0.5 (so you would go from 1.5 to 2.0 to 2.5). If that's true of your treadmill, then you'll want to do the following:

1. Warm up for 5 minutes at 3.2 mph.
2. For the first part of the workout, walk 2 minutes at 3.4 mph, 2 minutes at 3.5 mph, 2 minutes at 3.6 mph, and 2 minutes at 3.7 mph.
3. Then walk 5 minutes at 3.7 mph with a 3 incline, 2 minutes at 3.8 mph with a 3 incline, 5 minutes at 3.8 mph with a 4 incline, 2 minutes at 3.9 mph with a 4 incline, 5 minutes at 4 mph with a 4 incline, and then 2 minutes at 3.7 mph with no incline.
4. Cool down for 5 minutes, slowing to a stroll.

Inclines increase calorie burning significantly, much more so than walking faster. If walking isn't getting the weight off you, try hill climbing, stair climbing, or using a treadmill with an incline. You will burn far more calories than you do on flat ground.

Treadmill Intervals

The interval workout and the treadmill are a match made in fitness heaven because you can actually control both the speed and the incline of your walk, so you don't have to rely on RPE. As you know, there are two ways to increase the intensity of your intervals. First, you can go faster; second, you can go uphill. This workout does both! It really mixes it up, so you are constantly challenging your body, both aerobically and muscularly.

For your warmup, start to walk at a comfortable pace, but by the end of 5 minutes, get up to 3.5 mph at a level-1 incline. For the workout, do the following:

1. Walk 2 minutes at 3.9 mph with a 1 incline.
2. Walk 2 minutes at 3.5 mph with a 1 incline.
3. Walk 2 minutes at 3.5 mph with a 4 incline.
4. Walk 2 minutes at 3.5 mph with a 1 incline.
5. Walk 2 minutes at 4.0 mph with a 2 incline.
6. Walk 4 minutes at 3.5 mph with a 1 incline.
7. Walk 2 minutes at 3.5 mph with a 4 incline.
8. Walk 2 minutes at 3.5 mph with a 1 incline.
9. Walk 2 minutes at 4.0 mph with a 2 incline.
10. Walk 2 minutes at 3.5 mph with a 1 incline.
11. Walk 2 minutes at 3.8 mph with a 4 incline.
12. Walk 2 minutes at 3.5 mph with a 1 incline.
13. For your cooldown, walk for 5 minutes, returning the treadmill's settings to 3.0 mph with no incline.

Chapter 5
Swimming

Swimming is the gentlest of all aerobic activities. Unlike running, it doesn't have a negative effect on your bones and joints over time, and yet it makes a positive impact on your fitness and health. Water is healing, and swimming is especially recommended for those who want to prevent injury, use it for cross-training, are pregnant, are recovering from an injury, are suffering from joint or bone conditions, or are overweight and want to exercise in a weightless environment. You can build muscular strength and endurance, as well as improve flexibility and cardiovascular fitness, through swimming.

Why Swimming Is Great

The benefits of swimming are numerous. Swimming provides a cardiovascular workout without impact on your joints, is highly relaxing and meditative, and strengthens the major muscles. Also, swimming can be done indoors or out. Swimming is an aerobic, skill-oriented, stretching activity that improves nearly everything in your body except bone density (since it is not weight bearing). The skills and ability to swim are stored in your muscle memory, which means that when you take a break from it, you don't forget how to swim. It also means you can make improvements at any age.

If you already know how to swim but feel like you are treading water more than swimming, a few lessons can make the difference between frustration and enjoyment, as well as increase the effectiveness of your workouts. Your local fitness club or YMCA likely offers adult swimming lessons, and many cities offer swimming lessons through adult-education programs.

Recreational Swimming Versus Laps

Like walking, many people think they can swim the way they've always swum and call it a workout, but the truth is, to turn your swimming into an exercise program, you need to think slightly more scientifically.

The four competitive strokes are the crawl (freestyle), backstroke, breaststroke, and butterfly. Two strokes that are less strenuous and can provide a type of swimming rest are the sidestroke and elementary backstroke. Each stroke involves an upper shoulder or arm action, and a lower hip or leg-kick action with proper mechanics.

Freestyle is the most efficient stroke of them all, and the one most swimmers use for fitness. Butterfly is the most technically challenging and requires the most flexibility and coordination. Because it is the most physically demanding, it cannot be sustained for long periods of time. The backstroke also requires and improves flexibility and can feel like the greatest stretch of your life. Each arm reaches over and behind your head, enters the water at full extension above your head, and pulls down along the side of your body to your upper thigh. The breaststroke is fun to do and requires good timing. But if you have sore knees, you might avoid the breaststroke because of the lateral movement involved in the kick.

Swimming efficiently comes from practicing your technique. Even accomplished swimmers devote time to the basics. Swimming is considered to be 70 percent dependent on mechanical efficiency, and 30 percent on fitness ability. Efficient swimmers can stroke and glide quickly across the pool using as few as twelve strokes, versus the twenty or more it can take for less efficient swimmers. The power originates from the center of the body's mass, the hips.

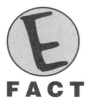

FACT

If you ever find yourself with an injury that keeps you from playing sports or doing your regular workout, give swimming a try. Depending on the injury, you can still usually swim. And even if you have a leg or arm injury, you can swim using paddles, fins, or a kickboard, allowing your noninjured parts to do the work.

Regardless of the stroke you choose, you want to create a productive glide, a smooth, continuous, advancing motion. Your reward is the fun, the feel, and ease of swimming like Flipper (the dolphin and TV star in the 1970s).

Another way to enjoy and enhance your swimming experience is to swim with the Masters. Masters swim is an organized group that meets to swim structured workouts made up of intervals and technique drills. Many communities that have a public recreational pool offer a Masters swim program. Masters groups meet several times a week at many locations and offer instruction, motivation, support, social interaction, and fun. Ask your local schools, community centers, and athletic clubs or gyms about Masters programs at their pools.

If you join a Masters team, you can compete if you're so inclined. Many groups train for competitions and swim meets. Racers compete against others of the same gender and similar age.

Lap Swimming

If you're going to make swimming a regular part of your exercise routine, you'll probably be going to a gym or public pool, so you'll be sharing the pool with others. To make this pleasant, rather than stressful, you'll need to follow the posted rules at your pool. For example, most pools post signs asking you to shower before entering the pool. Removing body oils, after-shave, perfume, and sweat before getting in the water helps keep the water cleaner and may help reduce the amount of chlorine used.

The one sign that is not typically posted but would be a healthy reminder is the "empty your bladder before swimming" sign. Some people are so excited, pressed for time, or both that they quickly change their clothes and head right into the pool, when suddenly their bladder begs for attention. Don't be one of them.

Most pools are either 25 meters, 25 yards, or 50 meters long. If you like to motivate yourself, you can learn the distance of one length of your pool. Then, by counting the number of lengths you've swum (and the time it takes), you can figure the distance swum and chart your progress. If it took you 45 minutes to swim a mile three months ago, and now you're doing it in 35 minutes, you know you have gotten faster and fitter.

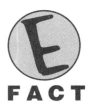

FACT

A lap refers to a sort of circuit, which in this case means you start at one end, reach the other end, and return to where you started. A lap is typically 50 yards, 50 meters, or 100 meters, depending on the pool. Swimming 1 mile in a 25-meter pool is the equivalent of swimming 65 lengths. Swimming 1 mile in a 25-yard pool is the equivalent of swimming 72 lengths. And finally, swimming 1 mile in a 50-meter pool is the equivalent of swimming 32.5 lengths.

Some pools have designated rules about lane sharing. If there is no sign posted and all the lanes are occupied, wait a few minutes and survey the situation. Find a lane where the swimmer or swimmers swim similarly to you. "Similar" can mean either stroke or speed. For example, if you plan to swim freestyle, it could be risky to share a lane with someone doing the backstroke or elementary backstroke. And if you are slower than the shark that is swimming in the same lane with you, it could be uncomfortable for both of you.

Unless the swimmer is swimming for time intervals, it is generally acceptable to interrupt and to ask to share the lane. If the swimmer is rigorously swimming intervals, wait until a rest or break in the workout to interrupt. Before you share the lane, ask the swimmer how he or she prefers to share the lane. If it is just the two of you, it is acceptable and oftentimes preferred to split the lane into left and right halves, claiming one side for each swimmer. For situations in which there are multiple swimmers in one lane, you swim in a counterclockwise direction. Think of it as traveling in the flow of vehicular traffic in the United States by staying to the right side. In this case, stay on the right side of the black line on the bottom of the pool.

Freestyle Swimming

Most swimmers use the freestyle stroke, in which you alternate between the left and right arms. Think of the hands as paddles. When the fingers are close together, the hand can pull the water more efficiently than when the fingers are spread open. Reach forward with a fully extended arm and use the hand to pull the water behind and beside your hip. As you pull, you will feel the water against the inside of your palm moving behind you, which propels you forward. Once the pulling arm is extended to the level of the upper thigh, it begins the recovery phase and repeats. This pulling action can be challenging for those with weak triceps (muscle on the back of the upper arm) and shoulders. The good news is that this stroke will strengthen them.

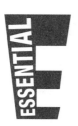

To avoid the dry, strawlike effect chlorine can have on your hair, wet your head in the shower before putting on your swim cap. Because hair can only absorb so much water, this prewetting helps the hair resist the chlorine.

When you use the freestyle stroke, your body rolls from side to side, causing a purposeful rotation, allowing the water to slip by. During this rotation, the gluteal muscles (your buttocks) move the center of your mass from side to side. The hips roll to a rhythm. The shoulders and arms are in sync with the hip rhythm and rotation. Good freestylers (and backstrokers) spend little time on their fronts or backs, and a lot of time rotating from side to side.

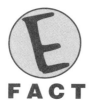

FACT

When you see swimmers splashing vigorously, they probably think their power comes from their kick, but that is not the case. The real purpose of the legs is to help maintain the ideal horizontal body position and to do so by kicking naturally, not forcefully.

You have two choices to make about breathing. You can choose to breathe on the same side each time or to alternate breathing between your left and right sides, called bilateral breathing. For same-side breathing, breathe every two (or other even number of) strokes, and for alternate breathing, breathe every three (or other odd number of) strokes. Most people are used to one-sided breathing and find it awkward to breathe on both sides. The benefits of bilateral breathing are that you can see other swimmers on either side, and that you will strengthen and stretch the muscles on both sides of your neck.

Let's say you decide to breathe only on your right side. As your right hand pulls and slides past your hip, your body rolls to your side so that you are facing the sidewall of the pool. Your head rolls with your body until your mouth clears the water. After you've taken your breath, roll back with your body until your head resumes its normal down position. Slowly release the air simultaneously through your nose and mouth until it is time to breathe again.

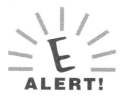

ALERT!

Good ol' dog paddling will keep you afloat, but if you watch a dog swim, you will see how quickly he fatigues. And so will you. Learn the other strokes, and leave the paddling to the pooch.

Swimming lengths continuously each time you swim can be boring. Work in some variety with intervals and drills using pull-buoys, paddles, fins, and a kickboard. An example would be to warm up for 5 to 10 minutes by swimming lengths and then vary the intensity level by grouping together numbers of lengths. For example, swim your warm-up and follow it with five sets of 50 meters at a moderate speed. After each set, take a short rest period, say 15 to 30 seconds, before starting the next set. After completing those five sets, you can do a few lengths of stroke and kicking drills. Then return to length swimming in sets of varying numbers. Remember to cool down when you are finished with the intensity part of your swim.

Swimming Equipment

While you can always head to the pool with just your suit, your workout will be that much more effective and comfortable if you buy a few pieces of equipment. Swimming equipment isn't as expensive as cycling gear, but it is just as helpful. For example, you might consider getting a wetsuit ($100–$200), bathing cap ($2–$12), goggles ($4–$27), earplugs ($2), noseplugs ($5), a kickboard ($15–$20), a pull-buoy ($15–$20), hand paddles ($15), and fins ($15–$40).

While you can usually try on goggles before you buy them, earplugs and noseplugs are, thankfully, not returnable. So you will have to risk a few dollars (they are inexpensive) to find the right fit. But having gear that fits well is worth it.

Swimsuits

Swimsuits are functionally designed for performance and allow for reduced drag and ease of movement in the water. With the many designs available, you can certainly find one that is attractive, supportive, and comfortable. When trying on a swimsuit, make sure the seams are comfortable around the legs (and for women, around the upper area, too). If the body of the suit is made of Lycra or spandex (as most are), it should feel slightly snug when you try it on because it is designed to expand slightly in the water for a comfortable fit. However, the seams and joints will not expand, even when wet, so make sure they are comfortable when dry.

Some of the best-looking suits can be literal pains in the rear (or front) if they don't fit you properly. So go for comfort, and if it does not feel good, try a different suit. Unless you are open to the idea of skinny-dipping and performing a bathing-suit-recovery exercise, save your skimpiest, least functional bathing briefs or bikini for leisurely water activities, and swim in your swimsuit. To enhance the lifespan of your swimsuit, rinse it out thoroughly in tap water after each use, and let it drip dry without wringing the life out of it. Chlorine, salt water, and lake residue can wear the fibers out prematurely. While you are at it, rinse your goggles too.

Wetsuits

Normal body temperature is 98.6 degrees, and the colder the water you swim in, the faster your body temperature is lowered. If the water temperature feels uncomfortably cool, consider using a wetsuit—not a scuba diver's wetsuit, but the type worn by triathletes. These kinds of wetsuits are made of a thinner, lighter, sleeker neoprene than those used for diving, and are designed to allow a full range of motion in the shoulders, as well as greater all-around unrestricted movement. Their effectiveness comes from capturing and reflecting your body temperature back to you, which keeps you warm. They also give you a slight feeling of buoyancy, which can be comforting.

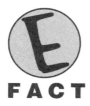

FACT

If you're swimming outside, remember the sun's reflection off the water is powerful, so use waterproof and sweatproof sunscreen (without these two capabilities, it won't stay on for long) on your face and all exposed parts of your body.

Wetsuits come in many styles. The warmest style has full-length arms and legs, and the coolest version is sleeveless and runs calf length. When trying on a wetsuit on dry land, it should fit very snugly; it will give just a bit once in the water. A definite must when using a wetsuit is to apply a lubricant around your neck so that turning and breathing doesn't cause your skin to chafe. Nonpetroleum lubricants such as BodyGlide are recommended, rather than petroleum-based products (petroleum jellies or gels) because the petroleum-based products can damage a wetsuit.

The Kickboard

You don't kick a kickboard; you kick *with* it. This Styrofoam board helps stabilize your upper body (you grasp the sides with your hands) so that you can practice your kick.

Training Paddles

These thin hand-sized hard plastic sheets with thick rubber semicircles through which you insert your fingers exaggerate awareness of your hand and shoulder positions and motions so that you get a feel for how your hands should be in the water. They keep you from slicing through the water and reinforce the correct technique of grabbing, or pulling and pushing, the water. They are also used to strengthen the arm and shoulder muscles by creating a larger surface area of resistance. The hand slips entirely through the larger rubber band, the middle finger slips under the smaller rubber band, and the paddle and the hand are as one unit.

The Swim Cap

The little swim cap does more than you might think. A swim cap protects your hair from total chlorine immersion, keeps your hair from clogging up the pool filters, helps keep your goggles in place, keeps your hair out of your face, and keeps your head warm. If your hair gets stuck in your regular latex swim cap, use a silicone cap. It is softer, and easier to put on and remove, and your hair will stay on your head, where it belongs. If regulating your temperature is a concern, use a latex cap in warmer environments, and silicone in colder ones.

The Pull-buoy

Placed between your thighs, the pull-buoy, a Styrofoam device, keeps your legs afloat, keeps your body in a horizontal position, and isolates your upper body so that you can practice your arm stroke technique.

Fins

Your feet slip inside fins. Kicking with fins will make you feel turbo powered in the water. It is hard to kick inefficiently with fins, but it is easy to kick too hard, so be careful. They put greater resistance on the quadriceps, hamstrings, and gluteal muscles, all of which strengthens your legs. They also create greater flexibility in the ankles, which makes for a better kicking motion.

Goggles

Goggles are used for seeing underwater and for keeping your eyes dry and out of the chlorine. The fit is very individual; however, even good goggles can fog up occasionally, so check that they are snug against your face but not so much that you get a headache or temporary tattoo. Try them on and see which ones cover your eye sockets best. Most goggles have an adjustable head strap, and some also have an adjustable nose bridge, which you can use to tailor the distance between the eyes. Occasionally, it is good to clean your goggles with soap and water. This removes the gradual buildup of facial oils that can cause the goggles to fog.

Earplugs and Noseplugs

Many people do not like putting their head in the water because the water seeps into their ears quicker than a mosquito slips into their house on a hot night. If you are one of them, a cheap pair of swimmer's earplugs is a quick fix. Some earplugs are made from plastic, and others from silicone, which, when warmed by your body heat, form to your ears. And if water up the nose and sinuses is irritating, use a noseplug. Once again, the fit and comfort is very individual.

Open-water Swimming

If you are privileged enough to live near an outdoor body of water, expand your swimming horizons to include aquatic workouts in open water. The freedom of swimming without walls, lines, and chlorine is very uplifting. Add to that the fun of swimming in a beautiful outdoor environment, and you are set for a peak experience. For safety reasons, it is best to swim accompanied either by other swimmers or by watercraft enthusiasts such as canoeists, kayakers, rowboaters, or surfers.

If you plan to be out in the water for a long time or on a hot day, your watercraft chaperone can carry drinking water or electrolyte-replacement fluids. Swimming, like all other aerobic activities, causes the body to lose fluids. But because you are in a cool fluid environment, it is nearly impossible to notice the sweat you produce. Add to that fluids lost from saliva and nasal secretions, and you can understand why you need to hydrate even while surrounded by water.

Stay abreast of the current weather and water conditions that will affect your safety, such as tides, undertow, strong waves (even in big lakes), and temperature. Your local parks or recreation department may have valuable information about the water that you plan to swim in.

Five Effective Swimming Programs

Many swim centers will have sample workouts that you can follow posted on the board near the pool. Do not be intimidated by the numbers and abbreviations. If you forget what they represent, ask someone to explain. Most swim instructions are given in yards or meters, not in lengths or laps.

The number in a half-parentheses, like (:30, is how much rest you get after each swim. For example, 6 x 100 (:30 means you are to swim 100 yards, rest 30 seconds, then repeat five times to do a total of six sets.

Normally the amount of rest per swim will limit your top-end speed on a workout, but that doesn't mean you should automatically go as fast as you can through the whole workout—and you shouldn't skip the rests. It is generally assumed that the stroke used is freestyle, unless it is specifically designated otherwise. Of course, you can apply your choice of strokes to the workout.

A good swim workout includes:

- a warm-up
- drilling (swimming-technique work, which can include speed work or stroke work)
- kicking practice

- pulling practice
- a main set of speed work
- a cooldown

You control how hard or fast you swim, and what swim strokes you want to use. The early parts of a workout should always be easy to moderate, and very deliberate. Use your best technique.

Skill-level Swims

Here are three simple workouts that you can follow over the course of 12 weeks. Start with the beginner-level program. After a month, move up to intermediate, and then try the advanced level after another month.

Beginner Workout	Intermediate Workout	Advanced Workout
Warm-up 1 × 100	Warm-up 1 × 300	Warm-up 1 × 500
4 × 50 S R:20	4 × 100 S R:15	10 × 100 (alternating 100 H R:20 with 100 E R:15)
8 × 25 S R:10	8 × 25 S	8 × 50 S
Cooldown 100 E	Cooldown 200 E	Cooldown 200 E
Total 600 yards	Total 1100 yards	Total 2100 yards

H = hard (very intense effort)   *E = easy (light effort)*

R:20 = rest 20 seconds between each exercise   *S = sprint*

Interval Swim

This swim includes speed work, which will improve your overall swimming speed, as well as give you a powerful cardio workout.

1 x 400	(:30
1 x 200	(:30
1 x 200	(:30
1 x 400	(:30
1 x 200	(:30
1 x 200	(:30

4 x 25	(:45 This is speed work.
1 x 200	(:45
1 x 200	(:45
1 x 200	(:45
1 x 200	(:45
1 x 200	(:45
1 x 100	(:45

Speed Workout

Try to do the middle swims with the longer rests fast to build speed.

2 x 500	(:60
2 x 100	(:10
2 x 100	(:10
1 x 50	(:30
4 x 25	(:45
1 x 50	(:30
4 x 50	(:60
1 x 100	(:60
4 x 50	(:60
1 x 100	(:60
4 x 50	(:60
1 x 100	(:60
4 x 50	(:60
1 x 100	(:60

Chapter 6

Biking

Remember how free you felt on your first set of wheels? Riding a bike is just plain fun, and it is not just for kids. Riding for fitness means you ride with intensity, specifically with speed and for time, or using hills to build strength. When you ride with intensity, bicycling is an aerobic activity that uses your hip, buttock, and thigh muscles. There is no pounding (as there is in running), and as long as you have a proper fit with your bike, you may feel as though you can ride forever.

Varieties of Biking

If biking piques your interest, you can enjoy road or mountain biking, or both! Road biking takes place on the road, and allows you to travel long distances with speed. Mountain biking is more technical and requires a sense of adventure and a secure sense of balance. Although the name implies it, mountain bike riding does not mean you are limited to riding on mountains. To ensure you have the proper frame size and fit on a bike, talk to your local bike-store expert or bike club. As far as seat positioning goes, your knees should have a slight bend (15 to 20 degrees) when you are in the down phase of the pedal stroke, and your hips should not sway from side to side when you pedal.

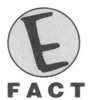

FACT

Riding a bike is a great way to get a hard workout in a short amount of time. You can ride indoors and out. Of course, riding outside will give you lots of fresh air, which will help you feel healthy and refreshed.

Of course, if you have never ridden a bike in your life and have no idea what it feels like, you need to go to a different book first. Once you can ride a bike and can balance safely, come back to this page. Now, for the rest of you, if you are riding again for the first time in a long time, do so in an area where you can relax and familiarize yourself with the gearing and braking systems. They may seem complicated at first, but once you understand how they work, you'll breeze right through them. Your body will initially have to adjust to cycling, so limit your first few rides to shorter periods of time and build up to longer rides gradually.

The pedal stroke is a smooth, circular motion. You want to not only push on the downstroke but also pull on the upstroke. This is hard to do on a bike that does not have toe clips or clipless pedals (an explanation of these terms follows shortly), but it is the correct bicycling motion.

Biking Technicalities

How do you know how hard to ride and which gears to use? The sport of bicycling has three major themes: efficiency, practicality, and self-sufficiency. Gearing is all about efficiency. You want to ride in the gear that will allow you to spin at a cadence that is comfortable yet taxing (here's the good ol' overload principle again). Spinning means pedaling with quick, even strokes at a comfortable and efficient cadence; this causes less fatigue in the legs than when pedaling at a lower cadence in a more strenuous gear. To spin, the selected gear has to be at a tension that allows you to push the crank (what the pedals are attached to) without straining. Cadence refers to the rhythm and number of revolutions per minute that you turn the crank. To help you visualize this: serious cyclists spin at 90 to 110 rpms, and recreational riders spin at roughly 70 to 90 rpms. Cadence will vary depending upon many conditions, such as whether you are riding on a smooth road or rugged trail, or up or down a hill.

The beauty of thinking about your cadence and spinning is that it keeps you from pushing a gear too hard, and that helps you avoid straining your muscles and other injuries. Once again, more is not always better.

Mountain Bikes

Mountain bikes allow you to ride on a wide variety of surfaces, including grass, dirt, rock, puddles, and paved roads. Mountain bikes are bigger, heavier, and more stable than road bikes, and at rest are more comfortable than road bikes. However, when you are riding a mountain bike up or down a dirt path, and over rocks or tree roots, comfort becomes a relative term. Mountain bikes have three chain rings (for gearing) and numerous gearing options that make it possible to ride through all types of challenges. The wheels and tires are larger than on any other type of bike in order to tackle the variety of terrain. Mountain bikes even come equipped with shock absorbers to help absorb some of the impact from riding over rough areas.

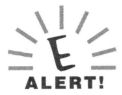

ALERT!

Knowledge of how to remedy a flat is important. You'll need to always bring a patch kit with you, which can be kept inside your saddlebag. Having the equipment with you can make the difference between having a fun experience or a disappointing one. The last thing you want to do is walk your bike home after you've already ridden for a few miles.

Hybrid Bikes

Hybrid bikes are a combination of mountain bikes and road bikes. They are best for those who prefer to ride on roads (great for commuting) but want greater stability and comfort than what road bikes offer. Hybrids are slower than road bikes and not nearly sturdy enough for serious mountain biking. They are heavier than road bikes but not as bulky or as heavy as mountain bikes.

Road Bikes

Road bikes are made from various grades of steel, aluminum, carbon fiber, and titanium. Generally, the lighter yet stronger materials command the heftier prices. *Components* is the term used to describe everything but the frame; it includes the brakes, shifters, derailleurs (front and rear), chain, chain rings, and cogs. Higher-priced components deliver a smoother, lighter, more reliable, more efficient, and more durable riding experience than lower-priced components.

Bike Equipment and Parts

Cycling is very much a sport dependent on equipment. The type of bike you have and its parts greatly influences how fast you'll go and how efficient your ride will be. If you're struggling to go fast because your bike isn't streamlined or appropriately sized, then you won't get the most muscular and cardiovascular benefit. Your ride should be challenging because of the course, not because your bike is old or broken down.

Aerobars

Necessity is the mother of invention, and that is exactly how aerobars came to be born. Since drafting (following closely behind another rider to avoid wind resistance) is not allowed in triathlons, triathletes and bike manufacturers came up with a legal way to cut down on wind resistance. Aerobars are U-shaped handlebars (or a handlebar extension device) that position riders more aerodynamically, with less air resistance. To use aerobars, the bicyclist leans forward and rests the forearms in the aerobar pads. In this position there is less air and wind resistance than in upright riding. They are best used on flat, smooth courses.

In addition to reducing wind drag, aerobars offer a greater level of comfort. They give the arms, shoulders, and hands a better feel as compared to riding down in the handlebar drops (the lower curling portion of the handlebar) or on top of the hood levers (the area on top of the brake levers). What is sacrificed in the aero position is dexterity and handling ability, but because riders can move freely in and out of the aero position as needed, it's still worth it to use aerobars. Aerobars can be used effectively on road, touring, and mountain bikes.

Toe Clips

Toe clips are metal or plastic pieces that partially cover the feet and help keep each foot attached to its pedal. After the rider inserts his foot into the toe clip, he tightens the toe strap to secure the foot in place. Toe clips keep the foot from coming off the pedal. They allow the rider to pedal efficiently because, with the foot secured on the pedal, the rider can pull up with forceful tension to create equal resistance through the entire circular range of motion of the pedal stroke. But toe clips have two major drawbacks. The first is that they can cause the feet to go numb. The second drawback is you need to remember to get out of them. To release a foot from a toe clip, the rider must loosen the toe strap first before pulling the foot up out of the cleat and out of the toe clip. Many riders either forget to loosen the strap, or can't react fast enough and fall over to the side, still attached to the bike at the pedal! Usually these falls happen at slow speed or when the rider is just barely moving, so the greatest injury is usually to the ego and not the body.

Clipless Pedals

These are safer, faster, and more comfortable! Clipless pedals mimic the downhill skiboot-binding system, yet with a sleeker, lighter, bicycle-specific adaptation. These funny-looking devices keep the cyclist's foot firmly in place on top of the pedal. Some even allow for wiggle room while the foot is attached to the pedal. To get into a clipless pedal, the rider steps into the cleat until a clicking sound is made, indicating that the pedal has received the cleat. To exit a clipless pedal, the rider simply pulls the foot up and out, away from the bike. The exiting, pulling action starts with leverage from rotating the heel out and continues with pull coming from the rest of the leg. The learning curve for getting in and out of clipless pedals is short, and cyclists can easily practice on the bike without worrying about injuring themselves. Once mastered, cyclists enjoy the freedom and strength they get from using clipless pedals.

Clipless pedals provide for efficient, comfortable pedaling because the rider's foot, shoe, and cleat are securely attached to the pedal. The clipless system makes getting the feet in and out of the pedal easier and safer than with a traditional toe-clip system.

Helmet

Absolutely, positively wear one. Even if you are an experienced rider, you can't control the other entities that could force you off your bike unexpectedly. Hard shell ANSI or Snell-approved helmets are recommended, and when it comes to quality, you do not want to skimp here. Most helmets are designed as one-crash helmets. That means they have a life of one crash. Some of the reputable companies will replace your helmet if you send the raked helmet to them along with your crash story. (Sounds odd at first, but after all, it is their business.) The biggest error made by novice cyclists is not wearing the helmet properly. It should fit snugly enough so that even before you tighten and secure the straps, it should firmly grasp your head without moving around. The helmet should rest toward the front of the forehead, should not slant up at an angle, and should cover the entire top of the head.

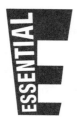

Even if your helmet has an attached visor, you'll still want to protect your eyes from the sun, wind, dirt, dust, and other airborne particles by wearing sunglasses. Sport-style glasses are designed to be lightweight and somewhat flexible. This means they will be comfortable even after many hours of wearing them. They are also highly durable, and as with most glasses, they will last a long time—as long as you keep track of them.

Shoes

If you are going to ride, you will want to get bicycling shoes. They have a very firm, inflexible bottom and a place for a cleat. The cleat provides added resistance against the pedal and adds strength to your pedal stroke. Shoes and cleats for mountain and road bikes are different, so make sure you specify which you want.

Gloves

These resemble the rough guys' knuckle covers in the old movies because the fingers are covered up only to the first set of knuckles. This allows for finger dexterity and ventilation. The padding on the inside reduces the friction that comes from prolonged riding or unexpected bouncing and jarring. Gloves help prevent blistering and reduce the overall stress in your hands. They protect your skin from road rash in the event of a fall. The least publicized (until now) but much appreciated role the glove fills is being a convenient handkerchief. You may wish you had a real handkerchief (remember necessity *is* the mother of invention), but . . . you won't. And for some reason, when people exercise, their noses have a tendency to run, the corners of their mouths get a residue or saliva buildup, or both occur. Enter the all-too-convenient glove or gloves that can easily wipe away these bodily responses and make you feel better while riding. In case you are wondering, bicycling gloves *are* washable.

Bike Shorts

Once you ride in biking shorts, you won't want to ride without them. That's because of the strategically placed seams and padding. The old-style shorts featured a chamois, soft pliable leather used for padding. But with today's high-tech fabrics, the leather chamois is nearly history. Synthetic chamois, as they are now known, will delight your personal parts with added support, comfort, and durability. Aside from the chamois, the shorts are made from a stretchy type of material such as Lycra, spandex, and Supplex, which offers support to the hips and leg muscles. The shorts also help to prevent chafing along the leg and groin area.

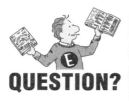

QUESTION?

Why are bike shorts usually black?
You are riding along and your chain comes off. You stop and easily put it back on the chain ring. Then you notice the new "artwork" on your hands and gloves made from black dirt and grease. Since you still don't have a handkerchief with you and you have to get the dirt off your hands, your shorts are the most logical place to rub the dirt off. Now, aren't you glad your shorts are black?

Biking Jerseys

Bicycling is all about being practical and self-sufficient. The bike jersey serves that purpose with its multipocketed back. Riders can fit most items in their back pockets, such as bananas (the cyclists' "meal in a peel"), sports foods, money, cell phones, identification, clothing, and many other items. All are within an arm's reach. Whereas experienced riders can reach behind them and retrieve the desired item from their pocket while riding and not lose control of the bike, novice riders may want to stop riding before retrieving these items. Bicycling jerseys are also designed for aerodynamic efficiency and safety. A proper fit is a snug yet comfortable fit. Wearing a baggy shirt while bicycling is dysfunctional and dangerous because it can get caught in your knees and even your chain (if you lean over or down).

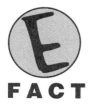

FACT

Biking isn't cheap. Here are some sample costs: bikes ($300–$1000), aerobar ($40+), a helmet ($30–$150), shoes ($60–$200), toe clips/strap ($6), gloves ($12–$30), clipless pedals ($50–$160), sunglasses ($40–$150), tires and tubes ($4–$50), biking shorts ($25–$80), a biking jersey ($21–$70), saddle bag ($6–$12), and a patch kit ($10).

Safe Riding

When you ride, you need to follow the rules of the road. Bicyclists must observe traffic signs and signals, and should use hand signals to alert others when turning or stopping, just as they would in cars. If you don't signal correctly, a car driving near you will not be aware of your intentions. Even when it appears that a driver is looking right at you, it is not safe to assume that you are seen and understood. Glare and other distractions play a large factor in drivers' inability to see a cyclist.

On that same note, when you ride on the street alongside parked cars, keep an eye out for drivers and passengers who are opening their car doors and don't see you coming.

It's also important to know bicycling etiquette. Communicate to your fellow cyclists. Common biking jargon includes calling out "on your left" to indicate when you are passing someone. Also, if cyclists are riding close behind you, it is good biking etiquette to point out debris on the road that they may not be able to see because they are close behind you, or "on your wheel."

Here are a few more details to keep in mind when stopping:

- The left-handed brake lever slows the front wheel; the right-handed brake lever slows the rear wheel.
- When you apply the front (left) brake, do so gently to avoid the force of your weight throwing you forward and overboard (or rather, over-bike).

- To slow down or stop, feather the brakes, which means alternating between squeezing and releasing them. It keeps you from being thrown off the bike, and it keeps your brakes from overheating and becoming less effective.

One more way to keep yourself safe when biking is to always make sure you are sufficiently hydrated. You can use two water bottles held in the bicycle's water-bottle cages. Most bikes have room for two cages. Or you can use a hands-free drinking system that you wear like a backpack. For really hot or humid days, you may want to use both bottles and a hands-free system. The advantage of using both is that you will be able to carry different fluids such as water and electrolyte replacements.

Indoor Cycling

If you like bicycling without the worries of the road, then stationary bicycling is for you. And if being mindless during exercise is your desire, you can best "slip away" more safely on a stationary bike than on other indoor aerobic equipment. There are computerized and noncomputerized bikes, and upright and recumbent bikes. Upright bikes position you as you would be on a traditional bike. Recumbent bikes position you in a semireclined position, which means the pedals and your feet are out in front of you. Recumbents were designed to support the lower back. If you suffer from "fanny fatigue" on an upright, you might want to try a recumbent. Neither style is better, so select that which is more comfortable for you.

Indoor Biking Is Still Biking

Even though stationary bikes may seem like pseudobikes, you still apply the concepts of spinning and cadence to them. Many bikes are equipped with a control panel that will display your cadence in rpms. With a cadence range in mind and a heart-rate monitor, you can familiarize yourself with what levels are aerobic and comfortable.

The biggest cycling error comes from pedaling at too high a resistance (either a high gear or setting). Exercise should challenge your body, but it is not supposed to hurt. Your goal is to spin with an intensity that elevates your heart rate but does not make you strain. The second error associated with bicycling is improper seat position. As mentioned previously, on any bike, you want to have a slight bend of the knee, about 15 to 20 degrees, when your leg is in the down position of the pedal stroke.

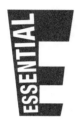

Before you get into cycling on a stationary bike, it's a good idea to be familiar with general stationary bike rpm ranges. This knowledge will help you gauge your performance and set goals for yourself. An athlete generally cycles at 90–110 rpms; a person who is very fit will do 80–90 rpms; and a decent workout registers around 70–80 rpms. If you're down around 60-70 rpms, you may want to double-check to be sure that the tension isn't set too high.

If the bike is mounted on a stand, stand on top of the support feet and then align the pubic bone over the seat. You should not wobble from side to side on the seat. Then get on the bike and pedal for a minute or two with your eyes closed. This will help you focus your attention on how biking at that seat height feels.

Spin Bikes

A spin bike is an indoor stationary bike that delivers the feel of an outdoor bike because of its stability, pedal action, and variable resistance. Spin classes are instructor-led group bicycling sessions that feature music, guided imagery, and varying levels of intensity. Although the popularity of these bikes comes partially from the class setting, you can ride them as you would any stationary bike when class is out of session. They have brought a new enthusiasm for indoor bicycling like never before. The pedal action is smooth and circular like that of a fine outdoor bike. The seat is narrow like a road bike, but a bit more forgiving. The seat also has adjustable settings for height, and for fore and aft positioning. A flywheel generates the resistance, and the bike's shifter allows you to vary the resistance. The shifter makes a slight click when the resistance is changed. The pedal is two sided; it allows you to use conventional exercise shoes on one side and cleated bicycle shoes on the other. Spin cycles do not have all the electronic feedback of other styles, so if you miss the spin class and want to combat boredom, bring along your headset. When you compare the feel of this bike to other stationary bikes, it is the closest to the real thing.

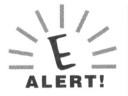
ALERT!

Do you feel tension in your knees, hips, or groin? Are you wishing you had two more legs to help you pedal? Are you pushing so hard with your legs that you wobble from side to side on the seat? Are you gripping the handlebars with the force of a rock climber? If you answer "yes" to any of the above, you could be straining on the stationary bike. Take it down a notch until you feel more comfortable.

Five Effective Biking Programs

There is nothing wrong with just taking a bike ride on a sunny day and not worrying about speed or resistance or mileage. However, as in walking, intensity is key, and another key part of training is knowing how effective your training is. You need to keep track of your mileage, as well as have a general idea of how hard you are working. You can use RPE (see page 11) or you can follow a regular interval program (using resistance on the bike or hills) to see how intense you can make your ride. In terms of distance, adding an inexpensive speedometer to your bike is the best way to keep track of your workouts, but you can also find the distance of a particular path with a car's odometer. If you know the distance you're biking, you can keep track of start and stop times to help you judge overall speed.

Your First Few Weeks of Training

Before you put yourself on a specific training program (whether you're on a bicycle outside, or a stationary cycle), take at least a week to work up to what is considered a moderate cycling day of 15 miles. Don't worry about time or speed on these rides. Take it easy and finish the full 15 miles, which can be done on a track, around your neighborhood, or on a trail (although it shouldn't be too hilly). The purpose of these rides is to gain and maintain basic cardiovascular fitness for cycling, as well as to get your muscles used to this new job.

After working up to the 15-mile moderate day, you can attempt an endurance day of double the mileage. Try to maintain the same pace you established during moderate days (in other words, it should take you double the time to do this ride). If you need to, slow down to make the full mileage.

After a few weeks at this level, try to do the 30 miles once a week. Or, if you work up to consistently higher mileage as part of your workout, do a double-the-mileage day once a week as part of your training.

Hills and Speed Intervals—Increasing Resistance

Now you need to find a trail (either plotted out for you or one you design) that includes at least one big hill. After you do a moderate day ride, go up the hill. Think of the ride down as recovery. Then, try to go up again. As your fitness improves, add more repeats. Hills increase your power and stamina.

If there are no hills around you, you can add intensity to your workouts with speed intervals. During a regular moderate day ride, pick a specific distance during which you will pedal faster. It could be, for example, a city block or even something as general as "up to that telephone pole." Or, if you have the odometer on your bike, you could pick a specific distance like a mile. During that interval, speed up to a sprint, pedaling as fast as you can. Start with one each ride, and then add more and longer sprints each time you ride. Sprint for one "lap," however long that distance is, and then slow down for a recovery lap, repeating the pattern as much as you want. Interval training and hill work improve overall speed, endurance, and your ability to recover, which are the keys to great fitness.

Interval Stationary Cycling

If you do your cycling workouts on a stationary bicycle, you still need to keep track of your mileage, speed, and resistance. Your resistance, of course, will come not from hills, but from the resistance you enter into your program.

The first thing you want to set a goal for is miles per hour, just as outdoor cyclists do. Then, if you want to add resistance, you'll increase the level number of your ride. This is the equivalent of adding hills.

Here is a sample interval stationary cycling program using speed as the interval. It assumes that you have worked up to a 15-mile ride, just like the beginner in the first workout.

Warm-up: 5 minutes at 11 mph.

Workout: 2 minutes at 15–18 mph; then 1 minute at 12 mph. Do this nine times.

Cooldown: 5 minutes from 11 mph to a slower speed.

Another option is to use resistance as your interval. So, for example, here's another sample program:

Warm-up: 5 minutes at 10 mph and level 2.

Workout: 2 minutes at 9–11 mph and level 4, alternating with 1 minute at 12–14 mph and level 2. Do this nine times.

Cooldown: 5 minutes, moving from 11 mph to a slower speed with 0 resistance.

These are fairly intense intervals. If you find they are too hard for you in the beginning, feel free to switch the intervals around. So, for example, your recovery time can be twice as long as the time for your intense interval. Eventually you'll work your way up to doing the program as it is written.

Spinning

Most of the time, the spinning teacher will lead the class, and you'll just follow her through the workout. However, if you want to do your own spinning workout, here is one that highlights what makes spinning great: high intensity coupled with a mind-body element.

This ride mimics a trip around part of San Francisco (including a killer hill). The visualization is the mind-body aspect. The best part? No traffic.

Warm-up: You're going to start in the Marina District. Start with zero resistance for 5 minutes.

One full turn: Stay that way for another 3 minutes.

Fast Flat: Do another two full turns and ride for the next 7 minutes around Fisherman's Wharf and the Ferry Buildings toward downtown. Try to cycle fairly quickly. This is a speed part of the ride.

Hill: You're going to go up to Coit Tower, which is an extraordinarily high hill (but not the steepest in the city and fortunately, you don't have to worry about turns). Raise your resistance three full turns (at least) and stand up to pedal. This should take 4 minutes.

Come down the hill: Lower your resistance two turns and pedal as fast as you can for 2 minutes.

Recover: Raise the resistance one turn and pedal at a moderate speed for 3 minutes.

Fast Flat: Let's go around downtown and up to Washington Square Park. Raise your resistance one turn and pedal quickly (but not as fast as you can) for 3 minutes.

Slight Incline: Raise your resistance two turns, and stand to pedal for 5 minutes.

Cooldown: Start to lower your resistance, getting it to zero within 5 minutes.

Make sure you stretch your legs after your ride.

Cross-training Stationary Cycling

There are few things as boring and as potentially monotonous as an endurance ride on a stationary bicycle. And if you're watching TV to make the ride go faster, chances are you won't be giving your all to the ride. To combat these problems, try the following workout, which is similar to workouts you would get in spinning classes that combine cycling with strength training or yoga or Pilates. These classes, which are very popular with regular spinners, build cardiovascular health as well as upper-body strength through resistance exercise, and increase lower-body strength through cycling. End the workout with an abs routine, and you'll have done a total body workout in one hour, including cardio.

Preparation: Place a body band near your bike, but not where you would step on it when you get off the bike.

Warm-up: Ride the bike for 5 minutes, gradually going from zero resistance to three full turns.

Slow climb: Do another full turn, and ride that way for 2 minutes. Then do two more full turns, stand up, and ride this way for 3 minutes.

Slow descent: Go down a full turn and sit down for 1 minute.

First strength interval: Get off the bike carefully and get your body band. Put the middle of the band under your foot and hold an end in each hand. Raise your arms in front of you to shoulder height for 30 reps.

Slow climb: Do another full turn, and ride that way for 2 minutes. Then do two other full turns, stand up, and ride this way for 3 minutes.

Slow descent: Go down a full turn, and sit down for 1 minute.

Second strength interval: Get off the bike carefully and get out your body band. Hold the band with each hand about 12 inches away from the center. Bring the band over your head and bring your arms out to your sides in a wide arc. Do this 30 times.

Slow climb: Do another full turn and ride that way for 2 minutes. Then, do two more full turns, stand up, and ride this way for 3 minutes.

Slow descent: Go down a full turn, and sit down for 1 minute.

Third strength interval: Put the center of the band under your foot and hold each end in your hand. Your arms should be straight down.

Bend your elbows and bring your hands toward each shoulder in a bicep curl. Do this thirty times.

Slow climb: Do another full turn, and ride that way for 2 minutes. Then, do two more full turns, stand up, and ride this way for 3 minutes.

Slow descent: Go down a full turn, and sit down for 1 minute.

Fourth strength interval: Put the center of the band under your foot, and hold each end in your hands. Bring the band and your arms behind you and over your head with straight arms. Now, bend your elbows and lower the band behind your head (this is an exercise called a French press). Do this thirty times. You need a very long band to do this. (If you don't have one, do a traditional triceps kickback with the band.)

Slow climb: Do another full turn, and ride that way for two minutes. Then, do 2 other full turns, stand up, and ride this way for 3 minutes.

Slow descent: Go down a full turn and sit down for 1 minute.

Fifth strength interval: Put the middle of the band across your chest and wrap the ends around your back, holding an end in each hand, palms facing up, hands near your chest, elbows slightly bent. Straighten your arms and bring them forward, away from your torso. Do this 30 times.

Cooldown: Get on your bike and pedal at a moderate pace and resistance, gradually going down to zero resistance. Get off the bike and stretch.

Chapter 7

Strength Training

Strength training (also called resistance training) develops the shape of your muscles. Here *shape* means the muscle has a definite outline; it's not all over the place. Strength training also develops and maintains muscular strength and endurance, develops muscle mass, stimulates bone density (which helps prevent osteoporosis), and reduces body fat.

Fit Bodies Have Definition

The word *definition* refers to the shapeliness of one's muscles. When your body has excess fat on it, it looks bulky and out of shape. Fat lacks definition, and it can be all over the place—your belly wobbles, your thighs are flabby, and your upper arms jiggle. In comparison, muscle has shape.

Women are often afraid of lifting weights because they think it's unladylike or not natural. However, unless you decide to spend hours and hours lifting very heavy weights, you will not get bulky. First of all, women do not have enough natural testosterone to produce major muscle size. And secondly, men build bulk only if they spend many hours each week lifting extremely heavy weights. As you will learn, there are many other ways to lift weights that will not produce such an effect.

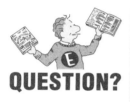

QUESTION?

Is it true that muscle weighs more than fat?
Yes, but not much more, and at the same time, muscle takes up less space than the same weight of fat, and muscle also burns more calories than fat. So, don't worry about muscle weight. It's good for you.

Strength training exercises isolate muscles and muscle groups, and, as mentioned previously, builds muscular strength and endurance. Muscular strength and endurance enable you to perform such tasks as carrying groceries and suitcases, taking out the trash, moving light boxes of papers or small pieces of furniture, picking up children or pets, or assisting older adults.

Improvements in muscular strength cause the body to burn more calories, even at rest.

Strength Training and Overload

Strength training exercises include weight training, calisthenics, and sometimes activities like yoga or ballet. We stimulate muscle growth by applying the overload principle, pushing your muscles a bit beyond what they are accustomed to. To strengthen muscles, we have the muscles experience resistance, or an opposing force. The terms *resistance training* and *strength training* are used interchangeably, and simply mean the process (just described) used to produce strength; the term *weight training* refers to using weight or weights as a form of resistance that produces gains in strength.

No Weights Required

A muscle gets stronger when it is stressed, i.e., when it is asked to work harder than it is used to. This occurs because the stress creates microscopic tears in the muscle, and then when the muscle is given time to rest afterward, it knits itself back together to become stronger and better than ever.

Muscle doesn't necessarily have to lift more weight to be challenged. If you lift your arm to the side right now and try to hold it up gracefully like a ballerina, you'll notice that after just a few seconds, your arm begins to feel tired. And that's because you don't normally hold your arm that way, so your arm is being "stressed."

If you continued to hold your arm up that way, oh, let's say, for 10 minutes a day, in about a week your arm would feel stronger, and it wouldn't be as difficult for you to repeat this exercise during the next week. Your arm would be stronger even though you didn't lift a weight.

The point is that you can build muscle without lifting weight. Ballerinas do it, gymnasts do it, and all kinds of other athletes become stronger in the very specific ways they challenge their muscles. For example, runners build strong legs; swimmers build strong backs, arms, and legs; and bowlers build one strong arm. Sounds silly, but it's true.

Strength-training Equipment

Again, the most common way for a person to build strength is to lift weights, specifically dumbbells, barbells, or weights on weight machines. But you can use medicine balls, elastic bands, and even soup cans or bottles of water to lift weight.

Dumbbells

Dumbbells are small weights. You typically can hold one in one hand, although you use two of them together so that you can have one in each hand to work your body evenly. Dumbbells can be anywhere from 1 pound to above 50, but most women stick to weights between 5 and 15 pounds. After that, it's pretty much easier to use either barbells or machines. Men go up to higher weights.

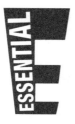

> Adjustable ankle weights wrap around your ankle and are secured by a Velcro strip. You change the workload by either adding or removing cylinder-shaped weights from the weight pockets. Ankle weights make leg exercises possible without machines. You can perform the leg extension exercise and the leg curl exercise on the exercise ball. The price of ankle weights ranges from $20 to $50.

Dumbbells are available at gyms, of course, but because they don't take up a lot of space, you can keep them in your house. They are infinitely versatile, allowing you to work almost any muscle. Also, because they start at very small weights and aren't that expensive, you can start light and pretty quickly increase the weight as you need to.

Using dumbbells is the easiest way for someone to build strength and lose weight. You can do the workout at your house, strengthen your whole body with just eight exercises, and see differences—seriously—with just a few workouts. In just two weeks, you'll really see a difference. (You'll find an all-dumbbell routine in Chapter 8.)

Bands

Think of a rubber band. If you pull it back between two fingers, you eventually get to a point where you can't stretch the rubber band anymore. Exercise bands, which are basically long strips of elastic of varying colors and tension levels, function as sources of resistance just as the rubber band does.

When you use an elastic band you put one end in your hand, or around a chair, or under your foot, and then pull the band. The other end is secure, so the band provides the resistance.

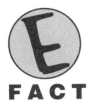

FACT

Your body will respond to bands in the same way it does to weights, i.e., you will build muscle and gain strength. Many people believe the bands are less likely to build bulk, but that isn't true. The reality is that unless you are a man using very heavy weights, then the muscular changes will be the same no matter what you use to build strength.

Bands come in a variety of resistance levels; some are hard to stretch and others are fairly easy. Each manufacturer uses a different color to signify the bands' resistance level. Some bands are flat and wide, while others are more like tubes with handles on the ends. The handles make them easier to hold.

Bands and tubes are not exact equivalents of weights, so you can't use a green tube and assume it is equal to 5 pounds, for example, or a dark blue band for 10 pounds.

Weights are much more exact than bands, but that doesn't mean they are more effective or better. It really is just a matter of choice and preference.

Bands are inexpensive and effective, easy to store, and, for many people, easier to use and less intimidating than weights. There is a total-body band workout in Chapter 8.

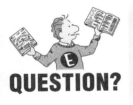

QUESTION?

Is it possible to spot reduce?
No. Spot reduction, the idea that you can just burn off the fat and sculpt the muscles in one area just the way you want to, is a myth. There is no guarantee that weight will come off where you want it to, or that your body will change with exercise in just the way you want it to. However, you can do specific resistance exercises to shape certain body parts, which will help you create the body as close as possible to the one of your dreams.

Medicine Balls

Medicine balls, which have been around since ancient Greece, are one of today's hottest fitness tools. They are now made from recycled materials, sand, and ground-up stones and bolts encased in leather or synthetic rubber. They weigh anywhere from 2 pounds to 35 pounds, and can be as small as a softball, bigger than a basketball, and in between. They cost between $15 and $150.

So how can this ball make you fit? As you throw and catch this round weight every which way, it builds muscles of the chest, stomach, back, arms, shoulder, legs, and hips. Medicine-ball exercises are fun and seem more like play, yet you can get aerobic exercise and build strength and flexibility. Having a partner is helpful, but you can use them alone too. You can exercise with them outdoors or indoors, but when indoors, make sure you have a clear space near you. One caution is to start with the lightweight balls; even they provide plenty of resistance.

Gym Versus Home

When you head to a gym, everything you might need for a workout is usually right there: dumbbells; weight machines; cardio equipment; aerobics, Spinning, yoga, and Pilates classes; and even a place to stretch. When you're at home, chances are you don't have a house full of weights and machines—not to mention a nearby trainer—allowing you to work each muscle exactly the way you should.

Gym workouts are not necessarily more effective than home workouts. Not everyone feels comfortable exercising in front of strangers, and if you're one of those people, then creating a home gym might guarantee you'll get your strength training in. Also, if time is an issue, keep in mind that it always takes time to get yourself to the gym.

Creating a Home Gym

A basic home gym requires an exercise ball, dumbbells, a step bench for step aerobics (which can double as a weight bench for women), a yoga mat, and some DVDs. Of course, you can spend from very little to quite a lot on creating a home gym. Here are some of your options:

Cost	Cardio	Strength	Core Strength/ Relax
Free	Walk/run	No-weight exercises	Yoga
Cheap	Jump rope	Dumbbells	Physio ball
Inexpensive	Step bench	Barbell	Pilates DVDs
Bells and whistles	Bicycle	Weight bench	Bosu ball
Top of the line	Treadmill	Weight machine	Pilates reformer

Even if you don't want to create an official home gym, it's a good idea to have at least some equipment and workout DVDs around for days when you can't get to the gym or go outside. For less than $100, you can always be ready to substitute a home workout for your regular walk, trip to the gym, or swim at the pool. And the benefits of the cross-training will help your overall fitness level.

High Weights/Low Reps Versus Low Weights/High Reps

Imagine two people. One is a man, the other a woman. They both stand in front of the free weights at their gym. They are both going to do overhead presses; in other words, they'll hold a dumbbell in each hand with a bent elbow at their shoulders, then straighten their arms and lift the weight over their heads.

The man holds a total of 30 pounds; the woman lifts 8. He does 8 repetitions, while the woman, who only has 4 pounds in each hand, does 18 repetitions. They are both tired at the end of their sets. Which one has done the correct workout?

Traditionally, men have lifted larger weights and done fewer reps for a combination of reasons. First, men are naturally stronger, and so they can lift heavier weights. Men also tend to want to make strength gains. For example, a man in a gym might want to become stronger, and thus hopes to eventually lift heavier weights as he progresses, while a woman simply wants to reshape her muscles and doesn't really care about being stronger per se.

Early in the research, women were advised to lift lighter weights and do more reps to make some sort of strength gain. But that really didn't work. The truth is, women should do the same number of reps and sets as men, and use a weight that works for them, which will be less than what men use simply because of basic muscle strength. For you to determine how much weight to use, you have to try out each exercise and see what weight will bring you to failure within the number of exercises you're doing. In terms of relative strength, the woman may make great gains—getting much stronger than she used to be—but she will never get big like a man, nor will she lift as much as a man. There are specific training programs using very heavy weights and low reps for body builders, but for your purposes, basic strength-training programs will work for both men and women.

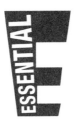

To create strength gains in your muscles, you need to work to failure, which means your muscle cannot do one more repetition. Failure doesn't mean that your muscle doesn't work anymore; it simply means that you have forced it to do as much work as it can do right now, and that it is ready to rest. And, as it rests, it rebuilds itself, thus getting stronger and shapelier.

Safety

Weight training is a safe activity, but it has the potential for danger because the equipment you're using weighs a lot. Drop a weight on your toe, and it will hurt! Twist the wrong way while holding a weight, and you will pull a muscle. Lift too much weight, and you'll hurt yourself so much that you won't be lifting for a while.

Stabilize your body weight and keep an erect back, not arching or swaying. Think of a cord coming out of the top of your head and pulling your entire spine erect. For most of the standing exercises, your feet should be shoulder-width apart. Rarely will an upright exercise call for your feet to be close together or touching each other. That is a sure way to lose balance.

As a general rule, you should exercise larger muscles before smaller ones. Smaller muscles help the larger muscles perform their work; if they are too exhausted from being worked out, the larger muscles will not be able to work as hard. Never weight train the same muscle group on two successive days. If you exercised your arms on Monday, do not work the arms again until Wednesday. Remember, this rest period is the time when muscle fibers repair and come back even stronger. If you want to strength train six days a week, then split up your routine so that rest and recovery can occur on different muscle groups.

Lift and Lower with Strength

There are two phases of exercise: the concentric and the eccentric. Those are technical terms for shortening and lengthening of muscles. When you bend your elbow to perform a biceps curl, you can see the muscle balling up or shortening; that is the concentric phase. When you slowly release the arm to your starting position, you are lengthening the muscle; that is the eccentric phase. Both phases work the muscles. During exercise, you want to exhibit control during both phases of the exercise, moving smoothly and slowly.

Take approximately four seconds to complete each phase of exercise. A common error is to work hard while performing the concentric, shortening phase of strength training, and then relaxing and letting gravity return the weight to the starting position. This is a waste of a strength-gaining opportunity, and it sets you up for injury by not balancing the strength gain.

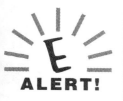

ALERT!

Start with lighter weight than you anticipate being able to lift, and if your form or posture suffers, lighten the load. Also be sure that you never hold your breath when strength training because that strains the heart. Instead, breathe deeply and smoothly as you lift and lower the weight. Exhale on the exertion.

When you lift weights, contract the muscles you're working, rather than passively allowing gravity to do the work for you. This actively stresses the muscle fibers, and your muscles will work more efficiently and respond more favorably.

Finally, make sure you exercise all of your muscle groups, with a few exercises per group. The groups you want to include are the back, chest, shoulders, triceps, biceps, abdominals, gluteals, hamstrings, quadriceps, and calves. But if that list overwhelms you and you find it impossible to fit all the groups into your life right now, then select one or two areas to get started; as you become familiar and comfortable with them, you can add others to your routine. Again, make sure that you don't exercise the same muscle group on two successive days.

When You're Sore

You should feel something in your muscles after you work out; typically, you will notice it most the morning after you exercise. Muscle soreness is actually a good sign. You want to get those sore muscles moving; when you do, you stimulate blood flow to the muscles, which facilitates recovery and growth. Think of the activity as massaging the muscle. But use your head. You don't want to work out sore muscles as hard as you can. Ease up on them a bit, and you will notice how, even after a few minutes of exercise, your sore muscles will actually feel better. Muscle soreness is also a healthy reminder to do some stretching and flexibility exercises.

Body Parts and Related Muscles

To make sure your resistance training is both effective and safe, you should be aware of which muscles correspond with what body parts. Consult the following images and read the descriptions of each part of the body.

Shoulders

Deltoids are the muscles that run over the tops of your arms. They are responsible for moving your upper arm in many directions.

The *rotator cuff* is a group of four muscles underneath your shoulder. They are used for throwing and catching, carrying, and reaching.

Back

The *trapezius* is the elongated diamond-shaped muscle that runs from your neck, across your shoulders, and down to the center of your back. It is used for most back functions, as well as lifting your arms out sideways to wave to someone.

The *latissimus dorsi* is the largest of your back muscles, and it goes from below your shoulders to your lower back. It is used for pulling. Strong lats help make sure your shoulders don't round forward.

Rhomboids are small, rhomboid-shaped (similar to rectangles) muscles underneath the *trapezius* at the center of your back. They are used to keep your shoulder blades together, which helps your posture.

Erector spinae muscles run the length of your spine, but you want to emphasize strengthening the lower segment of this muscle. All the spinae enable you to straighten your spine, to go from reclining or bending, and to stand or straighten your body.

Chest

Pectoralis are the main muscles of your chest. And yes, even if you have breasts, you have pectoralis muscles underneath. Activities that require you to push with your arms happen because of your pecs. They help to push a wheelchair, shopping cart, or lawn mower.

Upper Arm

Biceps are the two most famous muscles at the front of your arm. Any time you bend your elbow, you engage your biceps (e.g., when carrying small children or pets, and when lifting groceries).

Triceps are the three-headed muscles opposite of your biceps, on the back of the upper arm. They straighten your elbow and help out your pecs when you push something.

Forearm

There are many forearm muscles with too many names to mention here; think of them as your wrist muscles. Developing these helps prevent or alleviate symptoms of carpal tunnel syndrome and tennis elbow.

Abdominals

This set of four muscles allows you to bend at your waist, twist, and keep your torso stable. The abdominals (abs) and back muscles are neighbors, and when strong, they support your posture and back.

Rectus abdominis are the long, running muscles that start under your chest and end below your umbilicus (otherwise known as your navel or belly button).

Internal and external obliques run obliquely or diagonally down the sides of your *rectus abdominus*. These enable you to twist or bend at your side.

Transversus abdominis are the deepest of the four abdominal muscles. The transversus abdominis comes along for the ride when you exercise the other ab muscles. It is most active when you sneeze, cough, or exhale deeply.

Buttocks and Hips

Gluteus maximus, medius, and minimus are the largest muscles on your body. They are involved in nearly everything you do with your lower body, including walking, running, stepping, jumping, and getting up.

Legs

Quadriceps are the group of four muscles on the front of your thigh. These allow you to straighten your leg at the knee.

Hamstrings are the group of three muscles on the back of your thigh. These allow you to bend your leg at the knee.

Gastrocnemius and soleus are better known as your calf muscles. The gastroc is the rounded muscle at the back of your lower leg, and the soleus is just underneath. Women who wear high-heeled shoes may have some calf development (and chronic soreness) because the constant angled position of the foot causes these muscles to contract or tighten.

Tibialis anterior (shins) are on the front of your lower leg and go from just below your kneecap to the top of your ankles. These muscles allow you to extend or point your toes. They work in opposition to the calf muscles, so you want to keep them balanced.

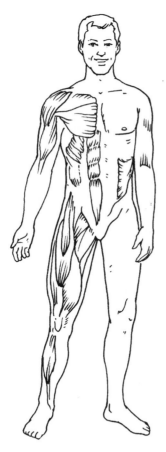

Our muscles, front view ▲

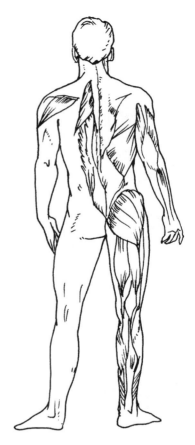

Our muscles, back view ▲

Chapter 8

Ten Effective Resistance Programs

Sports conditioning and fitness organizations recommend that you strength-train three to four times a week and change your strength-training routine every six weeks or so. They wouldn't recommend switching routines completely each time you exercise. Instead, pick one of these programs and do it for a few weeks. It will take a couple of sessions for you to figure out the right amount of weight to lift and how many reps you should do of each move. The way to stay strong isn't to just keep lifting heavier and heavier weights. Put some thought and planning into your program.

8

Drop-down Sets

A workout with drop-down sets (also called drop sets) is a great way to build strength and keep your workouts interesting. You'll start with a weight that's a little heavier than what you're used to—say 8 pounds for a biceps curl, for example—and then once that weight is too heavy after a few reps, you'll go back down to your usual weight, which might be 5 pounds in this case.

If you want to try drop-down sets, write down the exercises you want to do for each muscle group, and then try each exercise with a slightly heavier weight than what you're used to. You can even do drop-down sets with weight machines (this workout program combines free weights and machines). If you sit down, for example, on a leg-extension machine and you typically use 45 pounds, you can start by using 55 pounds, then drop down after the weight gets too heavy. And you can mix machines and dumbbells if you want, too. And each exercise might have its own combination of reps.

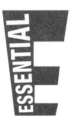

There are a number of ways and reasons to change your resistance program. First, your muscles get used to a program and stop responding as quickly to whatever exercises and weights you're using. Second, it's boring to just lift the same weights in the same pattern over and over. Third, no one exercise works all of the muscles in a muscle group completely, so changing exercises and routines means you're more likely to create balanced muscles and work most of the muscles.

Drop-down sets work because your body responds to the challenge of using the heavy weight, but you aren't overstressing your body by doing too many reps with that heavier weight. Also, by using the heavy weight first, you can do a few more reps in total since you are using the heavy weight before doing a set with the lighter weights.

Eventually, you'll do an entire set with the heavier weight. Once you get to that point, you have a choice: you can do a second set with the light weights, or you can pick out a heavier weight yet again and start the whole drop set process all over.

For example, let's look at the one-armed biceps curl:

Week One (three times a week):   3 reps with 8 lbs., 9 reps with 5 lbs.

Week Two (three times a week):   5 reps with 8 lbs., 7 reps with 5 lbs.

Week Three (three times a week): 7 reps with 8 lbs., 5 reps with 5 lbs.

Week Four (three times a week):   10 reps with 8 lbs., 2 reps with 5 lbs.

You could even, if you want, vary the weights more, such as:

Week Five (three times a week):   3 reps with 10 lbs., 3 reps with 8 lbs., 6 reps with 5 lbs.

So, on a Monday, your workout might look like this:

1. **One-armed bicep curl:**   5 reps/8 lbs.; 7 reps/5 lbs.
2. **Tricep kickback:**   7 reps/12 lbs.; 5 reps 10 lbs.
3. **Leg-extension machine:**   10 reps/45 lbs.; 2 reps/40 lbs.
4. **Leg-curl machine:**   8 reps/50 lbs.; 4 reps/45 lbs.
5. **Lat pulldown machine:**   10 reps/50 lbs.; 2 reps/45 lbs.
6. **Cable row:**   10 reps/35 lbs.; 2 reps/30 lbs.
7. **Squats with barbell or dumbbells:** 4 reps/20 lbs.; 8 reps/15 lbs.
8. **Chest press machine:**   10 reps/15 lbs.; 2 reps/12 lbs.
9. **Lateral raises with dumbbells:**   8 reps/10 lbs.; 4 reps/8 lbs.

One-armed Biceps Curls

Stand with your feet about hip distance apart, with a slight bend in your knees, your shoulders down, and your abs contracted. Hold a dumbbell in your right hand, with your palm facing out. Bend your elbow and bring your hand slowly up to your shoulder. Lower down. Do this for the full set of reps with the different weights, then switch to the other side.

Triceps Kickbacks

Stand with your feet about hip distance apart, with a slight bend in your knees, your shoulders down, and your abs contracted. Hold a dumbbell in your right hand. Put your left hand on your left thigh and bend forward from your hips, keeping your back straight and your hips in line with each other (i.e., don't tilt to one side). Bend your right elbow and bring your hand in near your shoulder. Then straighten your right arm so that your hand goes back to your hip. Return your hand to the start position. Do this for the full set of reps, then switch to the other side.

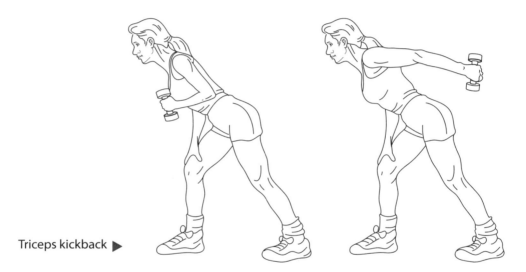

Triceps kickback ▶

Leg Extensions

Sit on a leg-extension machine, making sure your joints line up as directed by the instructions on the machine (use a back rest if necessary). Keeping your shoulders down, your abs contracted, and your back pressed gently into the pad, straighten your legs without locking your knees at the end of the move. Bend your knees, controlling the weight as you lower it. Do your reps following the drop-set schedule.

Leg Curls

Sit on a leg curl machine, making sure your joints line up as they should (use a back rest if necessary). Keep your shoulders down, your abs contracted, and your back pressed gently into the pad. Bend your knees, controlling the weight as you move your legs. Do your reps following the drop-set schedule.

Lat Pulldowns

Sit at a lat-pulldown machine, facing the weight stack. You might have to stand on the seat to grab the bar, but make sure your feet are flat on the floor when you do your reps. Lean back just a little as you bring the bar down to just above your chest, without hunching your shoulders. When you let the bar go up again, stay in control of it—don't let your arms straighten completely. Do your reps following the drop-set schedule.

Cable Row

Sit on a cable-row machine with your knees gently bent, your shoulders relaxed, and your arms extended, but your elbows not locked. First contract the middle of your back, then without moving anything but your arms, bend your elbows and bring them behind your arms without raising your shoulders. Go back to the start position. Do your reps following the drop-set schedule.

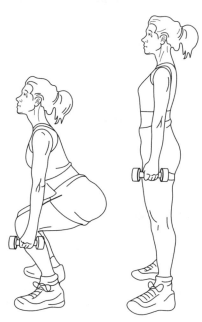

Squats ▲

Squats

Holding 10-pound dumbbells or a barbell at your shoulders, and keeping your feet hip distance apart, bend your knees and squat down slowly as if you're going down into a chair. Try to keep your weight back toward your heels. Stay down for a second, then come back up again, squeezing your butt cheeks together at the top. Do your reps following the drop-set schedule.

The Chest Press Machine

Lie on your back, with the bars at middle-chest level. Your wrists should be straight. Your lower back should be pressed gently into the seat. If you're short, feel free to put your feet on the bench. Your elbows should be bent at the start. Then straighten them, but be sure that you don't lock your elbows at the top of the move. Lower your arms back down. Do your reps following the drop-set schedule.

Lateral Raises

Stand with a dumbbell in each hand, feet hip distance apart. Start with your arms by your sides, elbows and knees in very slight bends. Raise your arms out to your sides without scrunching up your shoulders. Bring your arms back down to your sides. Do your reps following the drop-set schedule.

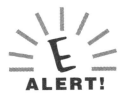

ALERT!

Hip distance apart isn't very wide. Put your fists together side by side (thumbs touching, pinkies farthest from each other), then place them on the floor. Put your feet on either side of your hands. That's hip distance (from hip bone to hip bone). If your hips appear much wider than that, it's most likely fat, not bone.

Of course, you have to write down a lot of information (reps, weights, and sets) with this type of program, but that will allow you to focus on each muscle you're working and give each exercise very specific attention to weight and reps.

20-minute Total Body Workout

When you're pressed for time, a total-body workout can help you accomplish a few things. First, it will build muscle and burn fat. Second, it can lift your spirits. Third, if you typically do a longer workout, a quick workout can challenge your muscles in new ways that will make it even more effective than your usual exercise routine.

The best way to do a total-body workout in a short amount of time is to exercise two muscles at once. These kinds of exercises are called compound exercises. Usually, for example, you will do a biceps curl to build that muscle, but with compound exercise, you might combine your biceps curl with a squat or a lunge, which allows you to work both your arms and your legs at the same time.

You can, of course, come up with your own compound exercises, but you need to remember (or, you'll soon discover) that these moves come with their own set of challenges. For one thing, you can't use weights that are as heavy because your energy and focus will be dispersed between the two muscle groups you are working. Secondly, there is a coordination element. It's not always easy to do a lunge with, for example, a lateral raise. Also, since you'll want to make this routine just as useful as your typical workout, it's best to do at least two sets to exhaust the muscle. Finally, you'll want to do a couple of full body-weight moves to fully challenge yourself. That said, the exercises are still effective and the routines can be fun and challenging. Here's a 20-minute total-body routine. Specific exercises are listed first, and details of the exercises, including the muscles that each exercise works and suggested weight amounts, follow.

1. Lunges with biceps curl
2. Row with triceps kickbacks
3. Squats with bent lateral raises
4. Chest press with hip lift
5. Pushups with leg lifts
6. Standing crunches
7. Standing twist crunches
8. Supermans

Lunges with Biceps Curl (Quadriceps and Biceps)

Hold 5- to 10-pound dumbbells in each hand, with your feet hip distance apart, your abs contracted, and your shoulders relaxed. Your arms should be by your sides. Step forward about three feet with your right foot. Bend both knees into a lunge. As you do this, bend both elbows into biceps curls. This requires a lot of balance (so you're also working your core muscles).

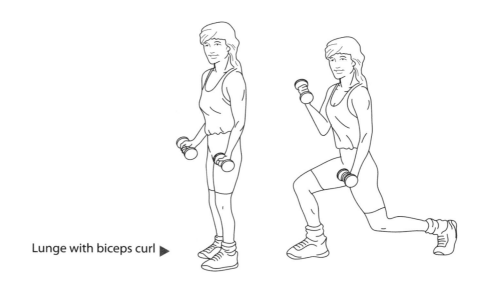

Lunge with biceps curl ▶

Step back, bringing your feet together and your arms down. Go to your left foot. Do this fifteen times on each side.

Row with Triceps Kickbacks (Back and Triceps)

Stand with your feet hip distance apart, your abs contracted, and your shoulders down. Hold a 10-pound dumbbell in each hand, arms by your side. Keeping your knees slightly bent, bend forward from your hips, letting your arms down straight under your shoulders, palms facing each other. Keeping your shoulders away from your ears, contract your back muscles, then bend your elbows as you squeeze your back muscles together. Straighten your elbows as you extend your arms without locking your elbows. Bend your elbows again, then straighten your arms and return to the start. Do this fifteen times.

Squats with Bent Lateral Raises (Glutes and Shoulders)

Stand with your feet hip distance apart, with 10-pound dumbbells in each hand, elbows bent, forearms parallel to the floor, palms facing each other. Keeping your shoulders away from your ears and your abs contracted, bend your knees and squat down. As you do this, raise your arms from the shoulders (kind of like wings). Bending down should take two counts; then hold at the bottom for two counts; and then come up, taking a final two counts. Do this fifteen times.

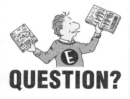

QUESTION?

I can't lift this much weight and do this many reps. How can I change the exercise?

No worries. You have two options. The first is to use lighter weights and try to do the full number of reps. The second is to use the heavier weight and do fewer reps. Both are fine, although using the heavier weight might help you build strength faster. But the most important thing is to do what you're most comfortable with, and what you'll stick with.

Chest Press with Hip Lift (Pecs and Butt/Hamstrings)

Lie on your back, with a 10-pound dumbbell in each hand at middle-chest level. Your wrists should be straight. Your elbows should be bent at the start on the floor, and your hands should be up in the air. Your knees should be bent, with your feet on the floor, and your shoulders away from your ears. Lift your hips up so that your torso and thighs are in a straight line from your knees to your head. As you do this, straighten your arms, but be sure that you don't lock your elbows at the top of the move. Lower your arms back down as you lower your hips. Do this fifteen times.

Pushups with Leg Lifts (Chest, Back, and Glutes)

Put your hands and knees on the floor, then straighten your legs so that you're balancing on your toes and hands. Your fingers should be facing forward, and the back of your neck should be long so that you're looking at the ground in front of your fingers. Be sure your body is long, too, from your heels to your head, with your abs contracted, hands directly under your shoulders, and shoulders pulled away from your ears. Lift

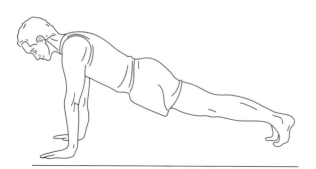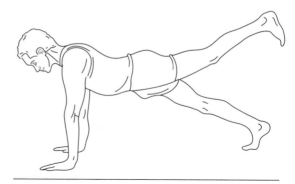

Pushup with leg lift ▲

your right leg without changing the straight line the rest of your body is in. Lower your right leg and raise your left. Then, bend your elbows and lower your body toward the floor without letting your abs sag down. Try to work your way up to fifteen of these.

Standing Crunches (Abs, Hip flexors, and Quadriceps)

Stand with your feet hip-distance apart, your shoulders away from your ears, no weights in your hands, abs contracted. Bring your arms up so that your hands are at ear height and your elbows are out to the side, as if you're doing a crunch on the ground. Keeping your abs contracted, bring your right knee up toward your chest as you bring your upper body down to meet it. Come back to the start position and repeat with the left knee. Do fifteen on each side.

Standing Twist Crunches (Obliques, Hip Flexors, and Quadriceps)

Stand with your feet hip–distance apart, your shoulders away from your ears, no weights in your hands, and your abs contracted. Bring your arms up so that your hands are at ear height and your elbows are out to the side, as if you're doing a crunch on the ground. Keeping your abs contracted, bring your right knee up toward your left shoulder as you twist your upper body down to meet it. Come back to the start position and repeat with the left knee. Do fifteen on each side.

Supermans (Back)

Lie with your stomach on the floor, with your arms out straight in front of you, legs straight behind you, facing the floor (if you're uncomfortable with this, put a folded towel under your forehead). On an inhale, raise your arms and legs just a few inches above the floor. On an exhale, come down. Repeat up to fifteen times.

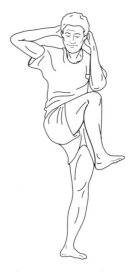

Standing twist crunch ▲

Machines at the Gym

Most gyms post a circuit that you can follow that is composed of one brand of machines, such as Cybex or Life Fitness. There is a machine for every body part, and the machines are placed in a row. All you have to do is follow the machines, right on down the line. This is a great way to get used to using machines. If you haven't lifted weights before, you'll really see and feel a difference in your body within two weeks. The order of the machines is something like this:

- Leg extension
- Leg curl
- Leg press
- Chest press
- Shoulder press
- Bicep curl
- Tricep kickback
- Lat pulldown
- Cable row
- Abdominal crunch
- Back extension

Dumbbells and Bands

Dumbbells, like everything else, have their pros and cons. They are easy to use and easy to store. However, you can't really lift a whole lot of weight with them. Working with dumbbells requires the rest of your body to remain strong and centered while you exercise, which is a strengthening benefit in itself. On the negative side, the fact that the rest of your body is working while you exercise a muscle means that muscle isn't doing all the work it could.

A lot of exercises can be done with bands instead of dumbells and bands. As you read in Chapter 7, bands are an inexpensive alternative, and many people find them easier to use than dumbbells. The following program is an all-over body routine with dumbbells and bands that focuses on one muscle—or muscle group—at a time. You'll need 5-, 8-, and or 10-pound dumbbells as well as bands, at least, to do this program effectively. Choose the weight size that suits your fitness level. You'll find more information on bands on pages 90-91. The specific exercises are listed first, with details of each exercise following:

1. Lunges with weights
2. Squats with weights
3. Plies with weights
4. Biceps curls
5. Tricep kickbacks
6. Flyes
7. Chest presses
8. Row
9. Shoulder presses
10. Front raises
11. Bent over flyes
12. Crunches
13. Oblique crunches
14. Leg raises

Lunges with Weights

Hold 5- to 10-pound dumbbells in each hand, with your feet hip distance apart, your abs contracted, and your shoulders relaxed. Your arms should be by your sides. Step forward about three feet with your right foot. Bend both knees into a lunge. Step back, bringing your feet together. Go to your left foot. Do this fifteen times on each side.

Squats with Weights

Stand with your feet hip distance apart, your shoulders away from your ears, your abs contracted, and your hands holding weights at your side. Bend your knees and come down until your thighs are parallel to the floor but your knees are not past your toes. Try to do this fifteen times.

Pliés with Weights

Start with your feet and legs spread out, toes turned out, butt tucked under, and your abs contracted (the second position in ballet). Hold the weights down between your legs. Now bend your knees without letting your butt sway out from under you. Come down until your thighs are parallel to the floor. Then slowly straighten your knees. Repeat fifteen times.

Biceps Curls

Make sure your feet are parallel to each other and hip width apart, with a band under both feet, and your hands holding each end of the band. Keep your shoulders relaxed and your arms down by your sides. On an exhale, bend your elbows and bring your hands toward your shoulders. You should feel tension in the band as you get to the top of the move. Lower your arms slowly. Repeat twelve times. Rest for 30 seconds and do a second set.

Triceps Kickbacks

Make sure your feet are parallel and hip width apart, with a band under both feet, and your hands holding each end of the band. Bend your knees a little and tilt forward from your hips, keeping your elbows bent and your hands by your shoulders. Now straighten your arms out behind you, bringing your hands to your hips. Bring them back to the start position. Repeat twelve times. Rest for 30 seconds and do a second set.

Flyes

Lie on your back with a band under your upper back, an end in each hand. Keeping your arms in a long line, bring your hands up and over your head, squeezing your chest muscles together when you get to the top. Return to the start. Repeat twelve times. Rest for 30 seconds and do a second set.

Chest Presses

Lie on your back, with a dumbbell in each hand. Your elbows should be bent at the start. Then, straighten them so that your arms come off the floor, but be sure that you don't lock your elbows at the top of the move. Lower your arms back down. Do your reps following the drop-down set schedule on page 101.

Row

Stand with your feet hip distance apart, with your abs contracted and your shoulders down. Hold a 10-pound dumbbell in each hand. Keeping your knees slightly bent, bend forward from your hips, letting your arms down straight under your shoulders, and your palms facing each other. Keeping your shoulders away from your ears, contract your back muscles, and then bend your elbows as you squeeze your back muscles together. Return to the start. Do this fifteen times.

Shoulder Presses

Stand with your feet together on the middle of a band, the ends of the band in each hand. Keep your abs contracted and your shoulders down. Now, raise your arms over your head, bringing the band up with your hands. Do not let your shoulders hunch near your ears. Return to the start. Do this fifteen times on each side.

Front Raises

Stand with your right foot about two feet in front of your left, toes facing forward. The middle of a band should be under your right foot, and an end of the band should be in each hand. Your shoulders should be relaxed; your torso tilted slightly forward, and your back flat. Your arms are down. On an exhale, raise your arms in front of your body to shoulder height. You should feel tension in the band as you get to the top of the move. Lower your arms slowly. Repeat twelve times. Rest for 30 seconds and do a second set.

Bent Over Flyes

Make sure your feet are parallel and hip width apart, with a band under both feet and your hands holding each end of the band. Bend your knees a little and tilt forward from your hips, then bring your arms down so they hang down. Now raise your arms up to the side, pulling the band up. Return to the start. Repeat twelve times. Rest for 30 seconds and do a second set.

Crunches

Lie down with your back pressed gently into the floor, your elbows bent, your hands behind your head, your shoulders away from your ears, your abs contracted, and your head and shoulders lifted off the floor. On an exhale, come up about six inches so that your eyes look in a diagonal at the ceiling. Come back down when you inhale without letting your head and shoulders go down to the floor. Repeat up to twenty times.

Oblique Crunches

Lie down with your back pressed gently into the floor, your elbows bent, your shoulders away from your ears, your abs contracted, and your head and shoulders lifted off the floor, and your right hand behind your head. Your right knee is bent, and your right foot is on the floor. Your left ankle is on your right knee, and your left knee is out to the side. Keep your right hand behind your head with your elbow bent, and your left arm on the floor. On an exhale, come up about six inches, and twist to your left knee without squeezing your torso. Come back down when you inhale without letting your head and shoulders go down to the floor. Repeat up to twenty times.

Leg Raises

Lie with your back on the floor; arms by your sides; legs up in the air, straight; and abs gently contracted. Slowly lift your hips and legs off the floor (you'll only be able to go about an inch or two), then lower back down. Do this slowly, and don't move your legs back and forth. Try to move straight up and down. Repeat up to twenty times.

Body Resistance

Before the 1970s and the advent of bodybuilding, almost all exercises relied on body weight for resistance. Oh, sure, a small percentage of people used medicine balls, barbells, and dumbbells for their workouts, but even dedicated exercisers relied on the most basic exercises, such as pushups, pull-ups, and sit-ups.

Once people began to understand more about how the human body became stronger, exercise machines were invented, and more exercises were designed for the use of those machines. But the fact is, body-resistance exercises (which use only the body and not weights) are, in many ways, the toughest moves around. In the first place, most of us can't lift more than our own bodies. So, for example, if you do a pull-up, which uses a number of muscles, including your biceps, and then if you do a biceps curl, chances are the resistance will be roughly the same, since the 8 or 10 pounds with the dumbbell will be equal to the percentage of your upper body weight that your bicep carries during the pull-up.

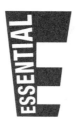

Even if doing a pull-up is roughly equivalent to doing a biceps curl with an 8 or 10-pound dumbbell, this doesn't mean free weights shouldn't have a role in your workout routine. Body resistance exercises are difficult, so doing bicep curls will help you build more strength so that you can do more pull-ups.

The following program comprises six exercises. If you try this program right now, chances are you will only be able to do one or two of each move—that's how hard they are. In fact, these exercises are such good indicators of true fitness that you might consider doing this program at least once or twice a week (it doesn't take long, especially if you aren't that strong and can only do one or two of each move) just to see how you progress. The individual exercises are listed first, with details of each exercise following:

1. Squat thrusts
2. Pull-ups (or pull-up variations)
3. Pushups
4. Walking lunges
5. Crunches
6. Supermans

Squat Thrusts

Stand with your feet hip distance apart, shoulders away from your ears, abs contracted, and hands on your hips. Bend your knees and come down into a full squat so that your butt is right on top of your heels, which are lifted off the floor. Bring your hands down to the floor as you get into this position, making sure they are secure, because in the very next second you're going to throw your legs out behind you and come into what looks like the top section of a pushup. Then come right back to the squat and stand up, bringing your hands to your hips. The squat thrust works your heart (because you're moving your limbs quickly), as well as your arms, chest, back, legs, and butt. Try to do this ten times, working your way up to fifty.

Pull-ups

With a pull-up bar in your doorway, put your hands on either side, palms facing toward you. Grasp the bar very securely. Pull yourself slowly up, bending your elbows and keeping your back and abs straight and contracted. Bring yourself up and over the bar. Then lower yourself down slowly. When you get to the bottom, don't lock your elbows. Try to work your way up to fifteen.

Pull-up Variations

Pull-ups are a great exercise, but you do need a bar to do them. If you don't have one, they're only about $20 at a sporting goods store. Once you get a bar, put it up in a doorway.

The other thing about pull-ups, though, is that they are tough! If you can't do them (and most women can't), here are a few other options:

- Put a bar or dowel across two chairs, and do the pull-up lying down on your back. You won't be lifting your full body weight, but you will still be exercising your upper body quite effectively.
- Try negative pull-ups. Put a chair under the bar so that when you stand on the chair the top of your head is level with the bar. Pull yourself up and bend your knees so that you're holding your weight at the top of the move (with your arms bent), then slowly straighten your arms and let your body go down slowly.

Pushups

Put your hands and knees on the floor, then straighten your legs so that you're balancing on your toes and hands. Your fingers should be facing forward, and the back of the neck should be long so that you're looking at the ground in front of your fingers. Be sure your body is long, too, from your heels to your head, and that your abs are contracted, your hands are directly under your shoulders, and your shoulders are pulled away from your ears. Bend your elbows and lower your body toward the floor without letting your abs sag down. Start with one and work your way up to twenty.

Walking Lunges

Stand with your feet a few inches apart, with your shoulders relaxed and your abs contracted. Step forward with your right foot and bend your left knee toward the ground as you also bend your right knee. As you come up, bring your left leg forward and do the lunge with the opposite leg. Go across the room and back, doing a total of twenty lunges on each leg.

Crunches

Lie down with your back pressed gently into the floor, your elbows bent, your hands behind your head, your shoulders away from your ears, your abs contracted, and your head and shoulders lifted off the floor. On an exhale, come up about six inches, eyes looking in a diagonal at the ceiling. Come back down when you inhale without letting your head and shoulders go down to the floor. Repeat up to twenty times.

Supermans

Lie with your stomach on the floor, arms out straight in front of you, legs straight behind you, and face the floor (if you're uncomfortable with this, put a folded towel under your forehead). On an inhale, raise your arms and legs just a few inches above the floor. On an exhale, come down. Repeat up to fifteen times.

Split Routines

With split routines, some body parts are worked on some days, while others are worked on other days. Therefore, some muscle groups rest while others work, and the working and resting times rotate. Serious strength-trainers do this kind of training so that they can exercise every day without inhibiting their progress because they know that a muscle grows when it is at rest.

One way to keep your total workout time from getting too long is to split up the body parts to exercise. The simplest way is to split up the body between upper and lower muscles. For example, on three days that fall every other day, you could exercise your back, chest, shoulders, triceps, and biceps. Then on the other three days (again, every other day), you could exercise your gluteals (buttocks), quadriceps, hamstrings, calves, and abdominals. There are other advanced split routines to use, and if you are interested, ask a trainer to advise you. This six-day-a-week program is merely an example, and not meant to overwhelm you. You could do the same program by exercising each muscle group once or twice a week.

Here is a sample split routine for upper and lower body:

Sunday	Monday	Tuesday	Wednesday	Thursday	Friday
Back	Glutes	Back	Glutes	Back	Glutes
Chest	Quads	Chest	Quads	Chest	Quads

Sunday	Monday	Tuesday	Wednesday	Thursday	Friday
Shoulders	Hamstrings	Shoulders	Hams	Shoulders	Hams
Triceps	Calves	Triceps	Calves	Triceps	Calves
Biceps	Abdominals	Biceps	Abs	Biceps	Abs

In this split routine, you are alternating the upper body and the lower body. Upper-body muscle groups include the back, chest, shoulders, and arms (triceps and biceps). Lower-body muscle groups include the gluteals, legs (quadriceps, hamstrings, and calves), and abdominals (actually, the abdominals can be worked on either day since they go from the upper to the lower parts of the body).

Ballet Strength

For ballet dancers, dance is not just about their legs, although, of course, their legs are extraordinary. It's their abs (flat and strong), their arms (thin and strong), and their backs (straight and strong). Ballerinas are thin, flat, and straight, but, more than anything else, they are strong. Their strength clearly doesn't come from weight lifting. Well, it does come from weight lifting, but it's not lifting dumbbells or barbells. Ballerinas lift their own weight and hold it, so much so that they can balance on a one-inch square of wood (in a ballet slipper) using just their first few toes.

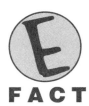

FACT

Ballerinas build their strength and skill through an endless repertoire of repetition. Rather than lifting weights, ballerinas build endurance and utilize core strength, which allows them to lift their body weight in extraordinary ways.

Ballerinas work on the flexibility as much as they work on strength, and, because of that, their bodies grow long as they grow strong, unlike bodybuilders or other athletes. The following program will help you strengthen your legs, back, and arms. When you do these moves, you'll want to focus on keeping your abs contracted, your shoulders down and pulled away from your ears, and your chest lifted. The individual moves are listed first, with details about each move following:

1. Demi pliés
2. Grand pliés
3. Tendus
4. Développés
5. Arabesques

Demi Pliés

Stand with your feet together, abs contracted, shoulders relaxed, and chest lifted. Keeping your heels together, move your feet so your toes face out. Your arms should be in front of your body so they form a circle, with your fingertips touching. Now, slowly bend your knees as you let your thighs separate. As you come down, your heels will rise. The bend in your legs should only be about 45 degrees. Come up, letting your thighs come together. Repeat up to twenty-five times.

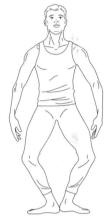

Demi plie ▲

Grand Pliés

Stand with your feet together but with the toes facing out. Then slide your right leg out to the side, setting down your foot when it's about three feet away from the other foot, and keeping your abs contracted. Bring your arms up so that your hands are touching and your arms form a circle, then open the circle without raising your shoulders until your arms are wide apart. This is second position. Now bend your knees without letting your butt sway out from under you. Come down until your thighs are parallel to the floor. Then slowly straighten your knees as you press your thighs toward each other. Repeat up to twenty-five times.

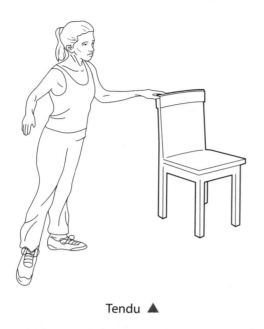

Tendu ▲

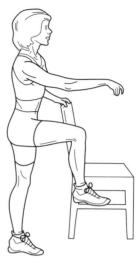

Développé ▲

Tendus

Stand with your feet together but with the toes facing out. Extend your right leg, letting your right toes slide along the floor, and stand strongly on your left leg. Slide your leg back in. Repeat this up to twenty-five times, then go to the left leg.

Développés

Stand with your feet together but your toes facing out, keeping your abs contracted and your shoulders down. Now, raise your right knee to a comfortable height (it doesn't have to be that high), and slowly straighten your leg at that height while keeping your toe pointed. Bend your knee again and repeat this up to twenty-five times without sagging into your left leg. Stand straight. Switch legs and repeat.

Arabesques

Stand with your feet together but your toes facing out. Slide your right foot out in front of you, straight, lift it up as high as you can (it won't be that high), touch your toe back down to the floor, and then raise your leg again.

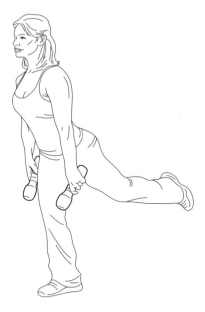

Arabesque ▲

Repeat this slowly twenty-five times. Then do the same to the back. You can lift your arms in front of you when you lift your leg behind you. Be sure to keep your abs contracted and your shoulders down throughout the exercise. Do this on the left side.

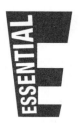

Ballerinas have beautiful arms. The main reason is the way they hold them in the air, which requires great strength in the triceps and upper back. If you try to hold your arms as a ballerina does, be sure to keep your shoulders down, your neck long, and the crown of your head toward the ceiling (not the chin). Lift your arms from the triceps rather than the biceps, so that the inner forearm slightly faces the floor. Extend the fingers gracefully.

5-minute Abs

Abs are many people's obsession. It's true, of course, that flat abs are synonymous with thinness and being in shape, but it's also true that abs are easily toned—if there isn't a layer of fat covering them up. So if you stick with this program and don't see a difference in your appearance, then it's time to focus on weight loss. The good news? Once you lose the weight, you'll be pleasantly surprised to see how strong and flat the muscles of your torso are. You only need to do this program every other day. And five minutes is actually plenty of time to see a difference. The individual exercises are listed first, with the details of each exercise following:

1. Crunches
2. Oblique crunches
3. Leg raises
4. Can cans

Crunches

Lie down with your back pressed gently into the floor, your elbows bent, your hands behind your head, your shoulders away from your ears, your abs contracted, and your head and shoulders lifted off the floor. On an exhale, come up about six inches, with your eyes looking in a diagonal at the ceiling. Come back down when you inhale without letting your head and shoulders go down to the floor. Repeat up to twenty times.

Oblique Crunches

Lie down with your back pressed gently into the floor, your elbows bent, your shoulders away from your ears, your abs contracted, and your head and shoulders lifted off the floor with your right hand. Your right knee should be bent, and your right foot should be on the floor. Your left ankle is on your right knee, and your left knee should be out to the side. Keep your right hand behind your head with your elbow bent, and your left arm on the floor. On an exhale, come up about six inches, and twist to your left knee without squeezing your torso. Come back down when you inhale without letting your head and shoulders go down to the floor. Repeat up to twenty times.

Leg Raises

Lie with your back on the floor, arms by your sides, legs up in the air, straight, abs gently contracted. Slowly lift your hips and legs off the floor (you'll only be able to go about an inch or two), then lower back down. Do this slowly and don't move your legs back and forth. Try to move straight up and down. Repeat up to twenty times.

Can Cans

Sit with your butt on the floor, hands behind you on the floor, torso long, shoulders away from your ears, knees bent, and toes on the floor. Lean back onto your hands without sagging. Stay long. Now, straighten your knees and extend your legs straight out in front of you. Bend your knees again, twist a bit to the right, and extend your legs to the right. Come back to the center and do the same to the left. Repeat a total of twenty times for all three directions.

10-minute Butt and Thigh

With all the sitting everyone does, the spread that used to be reserved for the few people who had desk jobs has now become something common even to men. And it's just so unattractive! These moves focus on all of the butt and thigh muscles so that if you do this routine you'll notice your lower half getting firmer and tighter. This routine combines the most effective moves from a number of disciplines, including ballet, strength training, and Pilates. If you want to supplement this workout with effective butt-burning cardio, try stair climbing, stair stepping, and spinning. The individual exercises are listed first, with details of each exercise following:

1. Demi pliés
2. Sumo squats
3. Sliding pliés
4. Leg extensions
5. Leg lifts

6. Hip lifts
7. Fireplugs

Demi Pliés

Stand with your heels together, toes out comfortably, abs contracted, shoulders down and relaxed, arms rounded in front of you, and fingertips together. Your inner thighs should be pulled together. Slowly bend your knees and allow your thighs to open without moving any other part of your body. Now, pull your thighs together as you straighten your leg. Repeat twenty times.

Sumo Squats

Keeping your toes turned out, widen your feet so that they are about three to four feet apart. Do not let your hips drop out behind you, and keep your torso straight, shoulders dropped down, and knees straight. Bend your knees and come into a deep squat, with you thighs parallel to the floor. Come up slowly, squeezing your thighs toward the center of your body. Do not let your butt sway out behind you. Repeat twenty times.

Sliding Pliés

Stand with your heels together, abs contracted, shoulders down and relaxed, arms rounded in front of you, and fingertips together. Your inner thighs should be pulled together. Slowly bend your knees and allow your thighs to open without moving any other part of your body. As you bend your knees, slide your right foot out to the right. When you are in deep plié, slide your left foot in toward your right and straighten your knees and pull your thighs together. Repeat to the right again. Repeat twenty times on each side.

Leg Extensions

Stand with your feet together, abs contracted, shoulders down and relaxed, and arms by your sides. Your legs should be pulled together. Lift your right knee without sinking into your left leg. Now, extend your right leg as high as you can (this might only be to knee height). Bend it again without putting your foot on the floor. Do this up to twenty times. Repeat on the left side.

Leg Lifts

Stand in front of a wall with your feet together, abs contracted, shoulders down and relaxed, and arms by your sides. Your legs should be pulled together. Put your hands on the wall, but don't lean into it. Keeping your right leg straight, put your right leg into a diagonal, toe on the floor behind you. Without changing your hips, lift your right leg up a few inches, then start the exercise: pulse your leg up twenty times from the lifted position. Lower your right leg and repeat with the left.

Hip Lifts

Lie with your back on the floor, knees bent, feet on the floor, and shoulders away from your ears. Keeping your knees together, lift your hips off the floor an inch without letting your back curve. Now start the exercise: lift your hips higher as you squeeze your butt together. Repeat up to twenty times.

Fireplugs

Get down on all fours on the floor. Keeping your right knee bent, lift it a little off the floor and then lift it to the right without straightening it or changing the level of your hips. Bring it down slowly. Do this twenty times and repeat on the other side.

Stay on all floors on the floor. Lift your right knee up a little and then straighten your leg out behind you as you lift it up on the diagonal. Repeat this twenty times, and then do it on the other side.

20-minute Band Workout

At first, band moves often feel easy because you aren't lifting any weight, but once you do a few reps, you'll begin to feel the way it tires out your muscles just like other resistance exercises. This is a great workout to do when you are traveling, because the band is an easy piece of equipment to bring along with you. Couple this with the no-equipment, body-weight series of exercises, and you'll see results fast. The individual exercises are listed first, with details about each exercise following:

1. Front raises
2. Lateral raises
3. Biceps curls
4. Tricep kickbacks
5. Flyes
6. Bent over flyes
7. Leg extensions
8. Woodchop

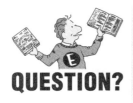

QUESTION?

What's the proper way to hold a band?
To hold a band properly, wrap the end around each hand so that the very end is under your thumb. Do not squeeze the end in your fist. Most of the time you will keep your thumbs up and your wrists straight.

Front Raises

Stand with your right foot about two feet in front of your left, toes facing forward. The middle of the band should be under your right foot, with an end of the band in each hand. Your shoulders are relaxed, your torso is tilted slightly forward, and your back is flat. Your arms are down. On an exhale, raise your arms in front of your body to shoulder height. You should feel tension in the band as you get to the top of the move. Lower your arms slowly. Repeat twelve times. Rest for 30 seconds and do a second set.

Lateral Raises

Make sure your feet are parallel and hip width apart, with the band under both feet and your hands holding each end of the band. Keep your shoulders relaxed, and your arms down by your sides. On an exhale, raise your arms out to your sides at shoulder height. You should feel tension in the band as you get to the top of the move. Lower your arms slowly. Repeat twelve times. Rest for 30 seconds and do a second set.

Biceps Curls

Make sure your feet are parallel and hip width apart, with the band under both feet and your hands holding each end of the band. Keep your shoulders relaxed, and your arms down by your sides. On an exhale, bend your elbows and bring your hands toward your shoulders. You should feel tension in the band as you get to the top of the move. Lower your arms slowly. Repeat twelve times. Rest for 30 seconds and do a second set.

Triceps Kickbacks

Make sure your feet are parallel and hip width apart, with the band under both feet and your hands holding each end of the band. Your elbows should be bent and your hands should be by your shoulders. Bend your knees a little and tilt forward from your hips. Now, straighten your arms out behind you, bringing your hands to your hips. Bring them back to the start position. Repeat twelve times. Rest for 30 seconds and do a second set.

Flyes

Lie on your back, with the band under your upper back, an end in each hand. Keeping your arms in a long line, bring your hands up and over your head, squeezing your chest muscles together when you get to the top. Return to the start. Repeat twelve times. Rest for 30 seconds and do a second set.

Bent Over Flyes

Make sure your feet are parallel and hip width apart, with the band under both feet and your hands holding each end of the band. Bend your knees a little and tilt forward from your hips, then bring your arms down so they hang. Now, raise your arms up to the side, pulling the band up. Return to the start. Repeat twelve times. Rest for 30 seconds and do a second set.

Leg Extensions

Lie on your back, with your lower back pressed gently to the floor and your legs up straight from your hips. Put the middle of the band over the bottom of your feet and hold each end in your hands, so the band goes down the length of your legs. Pull the band a bit to create some resistance, then lift your hips, pressing your feet toward the ceiling and against the band. Return to the start. Repeat twelve times. Rest for 30 seconds and do a second set.

Woodchop

Put the band over a top door hinge, then pull an end through the space between the door and the wall so that you're holding both ends. Stand with your hip near the doorjamb with both hands holding the band near your shoulder. Holding your torso very still, turn toward the door then twist down, bringing your hands to your opposite hip. Return to the start. Repeat twelve times, switch sides, then do a second set on each side.

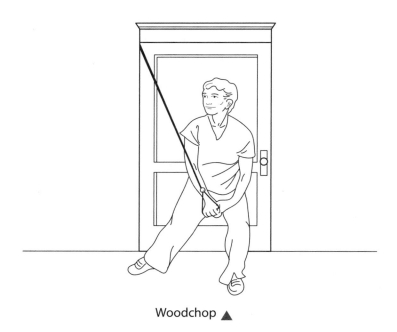

Woodchop ▲

Chapter 9
Core Strength

The core of your body is its middle, its very center, and it is what keeps your body in a straight up-and-down position. It includes all of the muscles of your torso—those in your back and abdominals. Ballet dancers have very strong cores, while people who sit too much have weak cores because they don't have to hold up their own bodies. When you think of the differences in these two shapes—even discounting the difference in body weight—you might use the words "long" and "elegant" for the dancer and the words "saggy" and "flabby" for the person with little core strength.

Creating a strong core immediately gives you the appearance and feeling of being thinner and leaner because you stand properly. It has been shown to reduce injuries in other athletic activities and to improve athletic skills. Football players, baseball players, surfers, and skiers all do core strength exercises.

The Muscles in Your Core

As mentioned previously, your core is made up of your abdominal muscles and your back muscles. Core strength reduces back pain because when your abdominal muscles are strong, your back has to do less work, and when it does have to work, it's strong enough to get the work done.

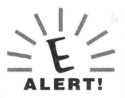

ALERT!

Because the *rectus abdominus* muscle is so long (running from below your ribs to your pelvis) you can work it in sections. Traditional crunches, for example, strengthen the top of the muscle, while leg lifts strengthen the bottom of the muscle.

Your abdominal and back muscles work together to keep your torso upright, so it's important to strengthen both groups. There are many ways to strengthen the core muscles, including movements that isolate one of the muscles in the group, or balance exercises, which force the muscles to work as a group. One example of a balance exercise is the plank pose. When you do a plank pose (like the up phase of a pushup), you are balancing on your toes and your hands. In order to remain straight and in a long angle from your toes to your head, your core muscles need to engage. If they don't, your belly will droop down, your back will sag, and you will rely on your arms and legs to try to hold your body up.

Other exercise styles that strengthen the core include swimming (because you are moving all of your limbs simultaneously), yoga (because you engage all of your muscles during each posture), and gymnastics (very similar to ballet in its balance requirement).

Over the past few years, more and more professional athletes, including football players and baseball players, have gotten interested in core-strength exercises because core strength is so important to overall athletic performance. When a football player has to reach up to catch a pass, he will do so with much less chance of injury if his core muscles are strong. When a baseball player has to crouch down to get a grounder, his chances of doing so with greater balance and more reach increase if he has a strong core.

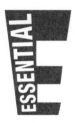

Another benefit to strong core muscles is that you can move your arms and legs more elegantly and with more ease than you can with weak core muscles. Ballet dancers (once again) have incredibly strong core muscles, which is one of the reasons they can move their limbs in a way that looks so effortless. It isn't effortless, of course, but they are able to balance and lift their legs so extensively because they rely on their core muscles to remain tall.

Back Strength

The back muscles become vulnerable to injury as we age for a variety of reasons, although the most common reason is misuse. We rely on our backs to do the majority of lifting and twisting in our lives, and yet we rarely take the time to strengthen them. Somehow, we think of our backs as sensitive, and yet rarely take the time to relax them. We force our backs into unhealthy, awkward positions (sitting in chairs, chief among them, but lying on couches and beds that are too soft are also problems), and then get frustrated when our backs aren't as strong as we would like. Even dedicated exercisers often ignore their backs because they can't see those muscles when they look in the mirror.

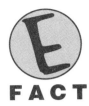

Humans are born with thirty-three separate vertebrae. By adulthood, we only have twenty-four, due to the fusion of the vertebrae in certain parts of the spine during normal development. Strengthening the muscles of the back helps keep the spinal column strong, too, which reduces the chance of back pain.

The Spinal Column

The spinal column and vertebrae protect the spinal cord, which provides communication to the brain, mobility, and sensation in the body through the complex interaction of bones, ligaments, muscle structures of the back, and the nerves that surround the spinal cord. The back is also the powerhouse for the entire body, supporting our trunks and making all of the movements of our head, arms, and legs possible.

The small muscles deep in the back play an important role in controlling the joints between the vertebrae of the spine. They steady the spinal column so that the long muscles of the back can use the spine as a lever when bending and twisting the torso. These muscles are therefore also important to posture.

Core Flexibility

One interesting piece of information personal trainers know and gym-goers don't is that gym injuries happen when people are picking up or putting down weights, not when they are doing exercise. The reason for this? Most people aren't flexible enough to properly move their weights around, even if they are strong enough to lift them. Twisting to put weights on the floor is hard for most of us, just as it is difficult for people to twist toward the backseat of their car or reach up high over their head.

Although strength is often thought to inhibit flexibility (strength shortens a muscle, making it difficult to stretch it) the reverse is true of a strong core, because it helps to be able to rely on the stability of your abs and back in order to lengthen and turn your limbs and torso. Think of ballerinas, gymnasts, and skaters. In general, they have the strongest cores of all athletes and, of all athletes, they are also the most flexible.

Pilates

The development of strong core muscles is the focus of Pilates, an exercise regimen developed by Joseph Pilates in the early part of the twentieth century. Pilates, a physical trainer, created these exercises when he worked in Europe after World War I helping to rehabilitate soldiers. His exercise system focused on strengthening the muscles the soldiers could use when their arms and legs were in traction.

Because the soldiers were in bed, Pilates used pulleys that moved their limbs for them as they contracted and strengthened their core muscles to initiate movement. This sounds complicated, but you can easily imitate what he did. First, lie on your back and press your lower back gently toward the floor. Now raise your arms and legs above the floor while still engaging your abs. You'll see how much strength it takes just to stay in this position for a few minutes. Pilates theorized that by strengthening the muscles of the back and front torso, he could help an injured man gain better use of all of his muscles and better control his entire body. In fact, Pilates was first called Contrology. Pilates moved to the United States and adapted his work for dancers, who found his techniques helped their strength and performance.

Today, Pilates students use Reformers, machines that have pulleys and a moving board, which require users to engage their core muscles as they use the resistance of the pulleys with their limbs to move their torso, which rests on the moving board. Reformers pretty much simulate what Pilates did with the soldiers who were confined to bed. But because Reformers are cumbersome and expensive, these moves have been adapted to floor exercises, sometimes called mat routines because they are done with a mat placed on the floor. They still require you to engage your core muscles and move your limbs, but you don't have the added resistance of pulleys. On the other hand, once you become very strong, you can use resistance bands to add a further challenge to your routine.

Exercise Balls

Another way to develop and strengthen core muscles is to work with an unstable environment, such as a physio ball or Bosu ball. This equipment forces your core muscles to remain activated and engaged for you to stay balanced. Let's say you are performing, for example, a leg lift. Traditionally you would do this exercise on the floor, which holds your entire body steady as you lift your leg up to strengthen your outer thigh. However, if you do the move with your torso draped over a physio ball (which could roll out from under you), then you must rely on your abdominals and back muscles to remain steady while you do the leg lift.

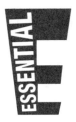

In another aspect of the mind-body connection, research has shown that exercise encourages creative thought because when one side of your brain is occupied with a repetitive chore, such as running or walking, then the more creative side of your brain is free to fly.

Exercise balls are easy to find in stores, and they're generally inexpensive—usually less than $25. They come deflated, but with a pump you can blow them back up. They come in a variety of sizes and colors, and you can do an extraordinary number of exercises on them and with them. They are great for beginners because they are fun, but they challenge even the most talented and skilled athletes, who are often able to actually stand on the ball while they work out, their core muscles are so strong.

Pilates Core Strength Program

This program doesn't take a lot of time, but it will benefit your health, your looks, and improve your performance in other sports and activities. Do this program three times a week. It should take about 15 minutes each time. When you do each move, pay special attention to the breathing instructions. When you inhale, make it a very slow, deep breath, and feel your body expand with the breath. When you exhale, do it slowly and feel your body get just a little smaller and more relaxed. The exercises are listed first, and more details about each move follow:

1. Toes in the water
2. Lean back with open arms
3. Swimming
4. Plank with leg extensions
5. Side plank

Toes in the Water

Lie with your back on the floor, knees bent, and shins in the air, parallel to the floor. Your lower back should be pressed gently toward the floor, with your arms by your sides and your shoulders away from your ears. Without releasing your abs, slowly drop your right foot toward the floor. You won't be able to get it to the floor, but bring it as far as you can go without losing the contraction in your abs. Bring it back up and repeat with your left foot. Then, try to drop both feet down. They won't go as far as one went. Repeat this whole sequence five times.

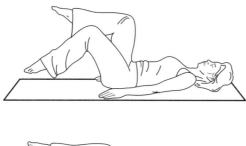

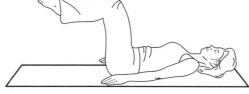

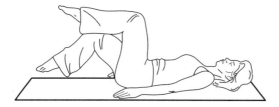

◀ Toes in the water

Lean Back with Open Arms

Sit on the ball, butt slightly forward from the top, knees bent, feet on the floor. Contract your abs, and keep your shoulders away from your ears as you bring your arms up in front of you to shoulder height in a circle, fingers close together, and lean back slightly. Now, turn to your right as you open your right arm out to the side and behind you. Come back to center and repeat to the left without sitting up. Come back to the center. Repeat the sequence five times on each side.

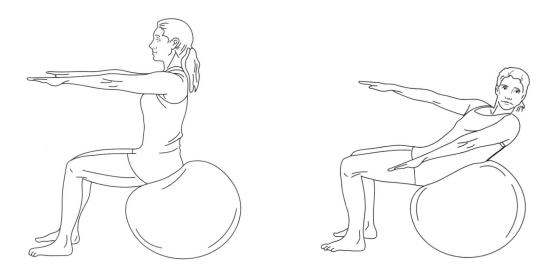

Lean back with open arms ▲

Swimming

Lie with your stomach on the floor, arms over your head, legs out behind you, and abs gently contracted. Keeping your neck long, lift your arms and legs just a little off the floor and start to "swim" with your arms and legs, fluttering them. Do this about thirty times.

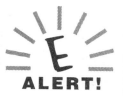

Try to stay conscious of your core muscles no matter what activity you are doing. To do this, simply tighten, without overly gripping, your abdominal muscles, bringing your lower ribs closer to your hip a fraction. You'll feel a contraction in your abdominals, and that alone will strengthen your core.

Plank with Leg Extensions

Start in a plank position, which looks like the up position of a pushup. Be sure your torso is long and flat, and your abs are contracted. Your arms are strong, but your elbows aren't locked. Now lift your right leg, toes pointing down. Don't lift your leg too high; it should just go high enough so that you feel a contraction in your butt, but your hips should stay level. Then bend your knee and bring it in toward your chest, once again without changing the line of your hips. Extend your right leg again and then lower your foot to the floor. Repeat on the left side and do this five times on each side.

Side Plank

This is an isometric exercise, which means you just hold the pose, rather than moving through it. It's tough, so here are three variations to try:

- **Hard Side Plank:** Put your right leg and your right elbow on the floor, keeping your left leg long, with your left foot on the floor, and your torso straight and long. Your left arm can be down along your side. Hold this position for two to five breaths.
- **Harder Side Plank:** Do the same position above, but balance on your right bent leg and your right hand. Hold for two to five breaths.
- **Hardest Side Plank:** Start in the plank position. Now, bring the right palm toward your left palm so it's on the floor just below the center of your chest. Now turn your body as you bring the outside of your right foot on the floor in line with the palm. Stack the left foot on top of the right, with the inner edges of the feet in contact. Press the

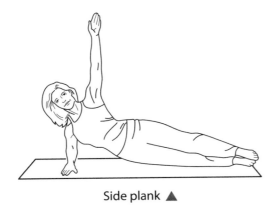

Side plank ▲

right hand down into the floor and lift the hips, making the legs and torso one straight line. Lift the left arm toward the ceiling, making the arms one straight line. Breathe and hold for two to five breaths. Come back to the plank position and repeat on the left.

Exercise Ball Core Strength Program

Just sitting on an exercise ball challenges your core because you have to stabilize your torso muscles in order to not roll off. These exercises, even when they aren't focusing on your core muscles, are challenging because you have to keep your balance as you do them. The exercises are listed first, and the details of each exercise follow:

1. Hip rolls with leg extension
2. Abdominal curl with leg extension
3. Single leg stretch
4. Criss cross

Hip Rolls with Leg Extension

Lie on the floor with the ball just in front of your butt, your right leg across the ball, your left leg extended up in the air, and your arms out from your sides at a slight angle on the floor. Be sure your back is gently against the floor. On an exhale, tilt your hips toward the left without letting your lower back lose contact with the floor. Let the ball roll with you and keep your left leg extended. On an inhale, return to the start position and roll to the other side. Repeat sixteen times, eight to each side.

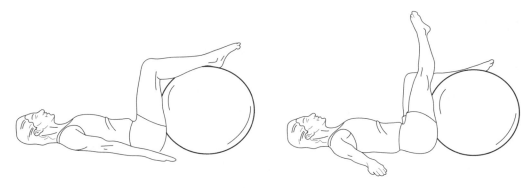

Hip roll with leg extension ▲

Abdominal Curl with Leg Extension

Lie on the floor, with your back pressed gently to the floor, and your hands behind your head, elbows out. The ball should be between your feet and lower legs, and your knees should be bent, with toes pointed. Your abs should be contracted, with your hips even on the floor. On an exhale, bring your head, neck, and shoulders off the floor as you straighten your legs. Keep your back gently pressed to the floor. You should feel this in your abs. On an inhale, come down slowly. Repeat sixteen times. You can do two sets if you want.

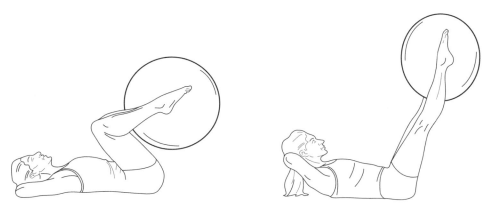

Abdominal curl with leg extension ▲

Single Leg Stretch

Lie on your back with the ball in your hands, above your torso. Press your lower back gently into the floor as you raise your legs to a 45-degree angle from your hips. Keeping your shoulders away from your ears, raise your head, neck, and shoulders off the floor. Bend your right knee and bring it in toward your chest. The ball should be just above your knee. Hold this position for two counts, then switch legs without moving your upper body and hips. Do this eight times on each leg.

Criss Cross

Lie on your back with the ball in your hands, above your torso. Press your lower back gently into the floor as you raise your legs to a 45-degree angle from your hips. Keeping your shoulders away from your ears, raise your head, neck, and shoulders off the floor. Bend your right knee and bring it in toward your chest. As you do this, twist toward your left slightly, bringing your hand and the ball down toward your left knee. Hold this position for two counts, come back to the start position, and then go to the other side. Do this eight times on each leg.

Chapter 10

Relaxation and Flexibility

Fitness is not only about pushing yourself; it is also about being in touch with your body. Being in touch with your body, or having a strong mind-body connection, means that you understand that your emotions, feelings, and thoughts are linked to how you feel and perform physically. It also means that, when you exercise, you bring your intellectual focus to your body, rather than letting your mind wander. This enables you to have a better workout and to achieve more meaningful and useful results.

The Benefits of Relaxing

Relaxation and flexibility are joined in the fitness world because the mind-body connection seems to best flourish in an atmosphere of gentle, slow movement. You can breathe deeply, slowing down your entire respiratory system and, in turn, soothe your nervous and parasympathetic nervous system.

Your nervous system is composed of the central nervous system or CNS (the brain and spinal cord) and the peripheral nervous system (other nerves and neurons that do not lie within the CNS). A further division is the sympathetic nervous system, which responds to impending danger or stress, and is responsible for the increase of one's heartbeat and blood pressure. The parasympathetic nervous system, on the other hand, is evident when a person is resting and feels relaxed, and is responsible for such things as the constriction of the pupils, the slowing of the heart, the dilation of the blood vessels, and the stimulation of the digestion.

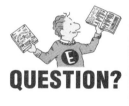

QUESTION?

I feel like I connect best with my body when I am participating in an intense activity. Is that possible?
Of course. Pushing your physical body can also push your emotional and intellectual boundaries. As mentioned previously, when one side of your brain is occupied in a repetitive motion, such as walking, running, or bicycling, the creative side of your brain is freed up to follow its thoughts and ideas. Also, changes in breathing patterns, whether it's slowing down your breath or increasing its intensity, can alter your emotions and your mood, which can lead to emotional growth and breakthroughs.

As mentioned previously, flexibility refers to range of motion, or the way your body parts can move around a joint. Flexibility level is somewhat genetic, i.e., some of us were born to be gymnasts and some weren't, but no matter what we drew in the genetic lottery, our level can always be improved (through exercise) or decreased (through disuse).

There are a number of ways to use exercise for relaxation and flexibility. The three mentioned here all use the connection between breath and movement, as well as a mindful awareness of what your body is doing. *Mindful* means to be conscious and aware of everything around you without judging or thinking about it. The most important thing you can do throughout all of these exercises is try to breathe fully and deeply. If you find the chatter in your head is taking away your focus and conversation, simply bring your focus back to your breath.

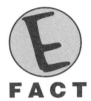

FACT

Stretching increases range of motion, which decreases chance of injury. It also improves posture and strengthens the core muscles of the body. Another great benefit of stretching is that it's calming and meditative. Concentrating on relaxing and stretching your muscles can rest both your mind and your body.

And speaking of focus, meditation, which is also described here, isn't a physical exercise (unless you have trouble sitting for a long time), but is instead a mental one. It won't help flexibility, but it does much to promote relaxation and concentration.

Yoga

Yoga has enjoyed enormous popularity in the last few years. Although it is a form of exercise dating back two thousand years, interest in its poses and accompanying practices, such as meditation and chanting, waned for generations, especially in its birthplace of India and the areas around the Himalayas. Now, however, westerners turn to yoga in all its varieties and styles. All yoga classes and yoga schools include *asanas,* or postures, that strengthen and relax the muscles. Almost all schools use the same poses, but some focus more on long, slow, deep breaths and slow movement, while others focus on movements that flow together with an accompanying breath.

Astanga, Bikram, Vinyasa, and western-style classes that are called power or hot yoga are the most vigorous forms. An astanga class includes postures that flow one to the other, so you never stop moving. Bikram includes twenty-six postures, each of which is performed twice, and always in a very hot room so that you sweat through the whole class. Each Bikram class is exactly the same, so you'll get better and better at specific poses over time. Vinyasa teachers vary the poses and flow sequences during each class.

Iyengar is a type of yoga that focuses on holding poses longer, and some Iyengar classes are restorative, meaning during all of the poses you'll be supported by blankets and pillows to allow your body to stretch more fully and relax more deeply.

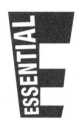

You don't need to bring anything when you take a yoga class, though you may want to have a water bottle if you're doing more vigorous yoga. Most classes will provide you with sticky mats (so you don't slip), and you'll be in bare feet. If you want to do yoga at home, you'll need a mat. They cost about $20 and are available in sporting goods stores and places like Target.

Whatever school of yoga you choose, you'll always want to link your breath with your movement. In other words, you'll focus on taking long, slow, deep breaths as you move, and you'll exhale with certain poses and inhale on other poses. The teacher tells you when it's best to breathe, but, of course, your breathing is up to you. The advice is just a way to help you get more out of your practice.

Tai Chi

Although tai chi is technically an ancient Chinese martial art, there is nothing martial about it really, although it is still artistic. Tai chi is made up of a series of flowing, slow movements that are connected with the breath. The individual movements are called *forms*, and each form often recalls an animal or something in nature, such as a tree or reed. Some form names include "Grasp the bird's tail" and "Wave hands like clouds." These names are evocative of the movement, which incorporate all the limbs and the breath.

Research on tai chi has found it to be helpful for mood disorders, such as anxiety and depression, as well as physical ailments, such arthritis and hypertension. Because you perform tai chi while standing and use your whole body, it can build muscular strength and slightly increase cardiovascular function. More than anything, though, tai chi is great for balance training, flexibility, and relaxation.

Posture and Relaxation

Are your shoulders hunched up close to your ears? Is your chin tilted up and your neck bent back? Or are you slumped forward, your spine looking like the letter "C"? Posture and physical tension go hand in hand. When you are tense, your body responds by tightening or contracting in some areas (the neck, shoulders, and lower back). At the same time, if you aren't standing properly or if you sit too much, your body gets uncomfortable and responds by feeling tense.

Stretching relaxes your physical body by relieving tightness in a muscle, but it also relieves psychological tension because when your physical body relaxes, so does your mind. Also, because we stretch slowly, we slow down our breath, which calms our nervous system. The best results for relaxation, though, come when we hold our bodies properly both when we stretch, and throughout our days. To do this, stay conscious of these three points:

- Drop your shoulders away from your ears.
- Your chin should be level with the floor, not dropped down toward your chest or tilted up, both of which crunch your neck.
- Keep your abdominal muscles gently contracted, that is, held in, as much as you can. Don't clench them, but don't let them sag out either. Letting them sag hurts your back and makes your posture unattractive.

Focusing on the breath during mind-body exercise keeps your mind from wandering and filling your head with chatter ("Do I look fat? Am I doing this right? What should I have for dinner?"). Connecting your movement to your breath is good for your body and your fitness. Many people don't pay attention to the way they breathe, and they breathe improperly (shallow breaths or fast breaths), which minimizes their body's ability to be strong and cardio-efficient. Breathing properly enhances your body's power and function.

Different exercise styles require—or at least suggest—different types of breathing. Traditional yogis, for example, breathe only through the nose, and many yogi practice a style of breathing called *ujjayi*, which focuses the breath on the back of the throat. And a Pilates teacher will have you focus on expanding your chest out to the sides while you perform his moves. But in general, to breathe properly and get you started before you learn more specific breathing styles, follow these instructions: Inhale through your nose, feeling the breath come in to your head and go down your throat and into your chest and belly. Your inhale should be so deep that your belly rises and you feel your body fill up with oxygen. Don't hold your breath, but let it flow through you.

Now, exhale by opening your mouth just a bit and letting the air drift slowly past your lips as you feel your body let go of the air and collapse gently without the oxygen filling it up.

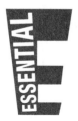

Be aware of the duration of your inhale and exhale. Your inhale can take anywhere from three to six seconds, and the exhale can take from three to nine seconds. You can, if you want, pause just very briefly at the end of each inhale and exhale.

Breathing deeply is perhaps the most relaxing thing you can do when you work out, or if you feel tense or nervous. It's a great thing to do when you're in a boring meeting. You can practice while you're watching TV or when you're in line somewhere. It's immediately beneficial and effective to your heart and nervous system.

Meditation

Perhaps there are two types of people: those who have experienced the scientifically proven benefits of meditation (they're the ones walking around with calm, happy smiles on their faces), and those who think it's some kind of freaky, chanting, flaky thing to do (they're the ones who are always wound up in a knot). The truth is, there are numerous ways of meditating; some include chanting, but most don't. And very few of them involve anything esoteric.

There are really two ways to meditate. The first is to focus on something, either visually or on your breath, and to allow that focus to take you out of your head so much that your breathing, heart rate, and nervous system relax. For example, if you think about your breath and begin to let go of other thoughts, then eventually you lose even your concentration on your breath, and your mind stops having racing thoughts.

The second way to meditate is to try to empty your mind. Try not to think about anything. This is often very hard for people, because we are always thinking. However, when you do this type of meditation, you simply sit and let go. Thoughts will occur to you, but you just let them pass. Don't ruminate on them or connect them to another thought.

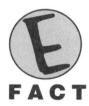

FACT

Meditation helps you learn to control your breathing and heart rate, which is useful during exercise, because as you become better at breathing, you can take deeper and more constructive breaths even while you're working out at a high intensity. Also, as you've learned, the true measure of fitness is recovery time and efficiency—how long it takes your heart to slow down after effort and how easily your heart responds to effort—and meditation helps both of those measures.

One of the best ways to experience the benefits of meditation is to do it for a just a minute. Right now, sit up, make sure your feet are supported (if you're in a chair, they should be on the floor), and bring your mental focus to the in and out of your breath.

As you do this, try to slow down both your inhale and your exhale, making your breaths deeper and longer. Bring your breath deep into your body and imagine it expanding so far that it fills all of you, even your fingertips and toes.

Continue breathing deeply and focusing on your breath. Some thoughts will come into your head, but just let them pass. Eventually you will feel your heart rate and breathing rate slow. If you get anxious or too self-aware, just stop and try again tomorrow. Continue this type of practice, eventually working your way up to ten minutes of meditation.

Stretching

We all stretch—lengthen parts of our bodies—naturally. We get up and put our hands behind our backs and push our pelvises out to reverse the curve our back has been in. We reach over our heads to lengthen our spines from sitting. Stretching, even if it's not a formal program, feels good and seems to relieve muscle tension.

Research has recently found that stretching briefly before a workout doesn't really prevent injuries as it was thought to, but stretching throughout the day is good for us. And stretching after a strength workout has actually been shown to promote strength gains.

Psychologically, stretching gives your mind some time to transition from one activity to another. If you're sitting and stand up to stretch, then it helps your body get ready to move. If you've been exercising and you stretch when you're done, this time gives you a minute to calm down and change your mental focus.

It's very important to look at stretching not as a challenge, as in "How far can I pull my leg to one side?" but as a treat for your body. That's because overstretching can hurt your body as much as any type of overtraining. You should also never bounce as you stretch. For example, let's say you're stretching the back of your upper leg, the hamstring muscle. To do this, you can put your leg up on a bench or step, and lean your torso over your leg. This lengthens your hamstring muscles, which is a stretch. You might not feel it, though, so you lean down further until you feel it. If you keep leaning and leaning or bouncing and bouncing so much that you're not paying attention to how the stretch feels, you could pull your muscle longer than it's able to go, which can rip or tear it.

Instead, use your breath to guide your stretch (just as you do during yoga and Pilates). As you exhale, stretch just a little more and, when you inhale, ease up on the stretch. Then, when you exhale again, stretch a little more. Following your breath will ensure that you don't overstretch and that you're not bouncing.

Five Effective Relaxation and Stretching Programs

Breathing deeply. Achieving calm and serenity. Loosening your tight muscles. It's rarely difficult to convince people to stretch because it just feels so good. And because it feels so good, lots of people think there's no physical benefit to stretching, but of course, that's not true. Each of these programs will end with you feeling calmer and more centered, with your mind and body connected, functioning as one.

Now, you can do these programs as often as you want and in any particular order. These routines won't stress your body in any way, so you don't need to rest or recover from them. All you need to do is enjoy.

Fifteen-minute Yoga Program

Just as there are a large number of yoga poses, or asanas, and variations on each of those poses, there are also an endless number of ways to put those postures together into sequences and routines. Like most yoga routines, this program focuses on connecting the breath with moves that will increase your flexibility in a slow, relaxing manner. This is a great routine for after work or before bed. Read it through a few times first so you can cover your eyes when necessary.

Mountain

Stand with feet pressed gently together, feeling all five toes and your heels on the floor. Pull your quadriceps up and away from your knees, contract your abs, and drop your shoulders down and back, away from your ears. This is Mountain pose. Now bring your palms up to cover your eyes and take three long, slow, deep breaths (inhale and exhale). When you feel centered, take your palms away from your eyes and lower your arms to your sides.

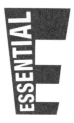

If, at any time, you feel yourself getting tense or self-conscious when you're practicing yoga, remind yourself to take a few breaths and focus on your slow inhale and exhale. This will help you relax both your mind and your body again.

Reed

Keeping your feet together and the rest of your body strong, raise your arms up, straight over your head, with your palms facing each other. Be sure to keep your shoulders down, not hunched up to your ears. Inhale and reach up with your torso, becoming longer. Then, on an exhale, reach your torso and arms to the right without leaning forward or back. Keep your feet planted and your abs contracted. Continue to breathe fully, allowing your body to move gently (like a reed in the wind) rather than trying to hold it still. On an inhale, come up to the start position and repeat to the left side. Come back to the start again. Lower your arms to your sides.

Forward Bend

On an inhale, bring your arms up and over your head, without hunching your shoulders up to your ears. Then on your exhale, roll forward, coming as far down as you can without pulling yourself down. Feel free to bend your knees a little. Bring your hands to your shins, feet, or to the floor next to you. Continue to breathe deeply for about five cycles (one inhale and exhale=one cycle). Your stretch will get deeper as you hold the pose.

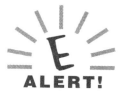

ALERT!

Forward bends, like some other yoga stretches, are very extreme. This move stretches your hamstrings and lower back. Give yourself permission to relax into the posture rather than forcing yourself into it, as you don't want to pull a muscle. Always focus on your breath, not how far you can go. If you can't breathe deeply and slowly, you're pushing yourself.

Standing Arch

Place your hands on your shins, feet, or on the floor next to your feet, and begin to straighten your torso so that it forms a right angle to your legs, which are straightening (but your knees aren't locked). You should look like a triangle from the side. Pull your shoulders away from your ears as you continue to reach forward with your head and torso, and press your feet into the floor as you press your butt away from your head and lift your hips out of your thighs. This is a true feeling of reaching in all directions. Hold for a few breath cycles.

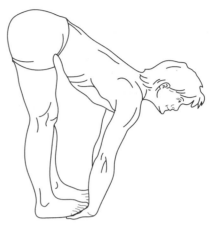

Standing arch ▲

Transition

Come back down to forward bend. Then let your hands and arms come out to the sides as you begin to stand up, keeping your hips gently tucked under and your abs contracted. Come to Mountain pose. Then come to the floor on all fours (knees and hands on the floor).

Cat/Dog

Start with your hands, knees, and shins on the floor. Your hands should be directly under your shoulders, and your knees should be directly under your hips, with the tops of your feet against the floor. Allow your back to feel natural. Your eyes should be looking at the floor, slightly past your hands. Now, on an inhale, turn your face up, and drop your shoulders away from your ears as you tilt your butt up, letting your back sway. This should take a couple of seconds, and you should really feel your hips and lower back release. When you are ready to exhale, turn your hips in the opposite direction and look down, letting your back go into a slow arch, like a hissing cat. The difference between the two moves should be extreme, but you should flow from each move in a slow and controlled manner. Do this five or six times, with long, deep breaths, eventually returning to the neutral position.

Downward Facing Dog

Turn your toes under and begin to press evenly into your palms and toes as you lift your butt up and straighten your knees. Make your torso straight and long, as if you're moving through your arms as you straighten your legs and lift your hips. You should look like a very strong and straight inverted V. Try to press your heels to the floor, and press down evenly on all of your fingers as you lift your hips high. Let your neck be relaxed. Hold this for five breath cycles and, as you breathe, try to both relax and be stronger in this pose.

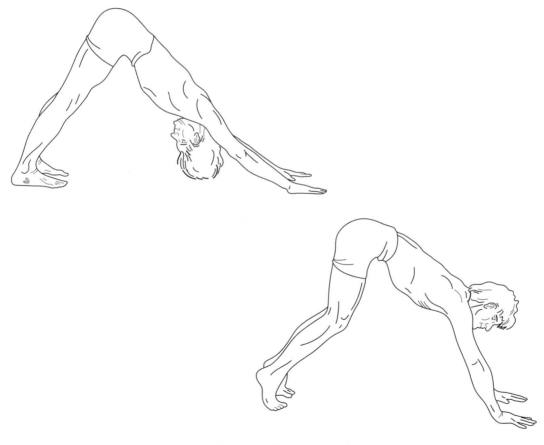

Downward facing dog ▲

Child's Pose

Come down to your belly on the floor, with your arms outstretched above your head and your legs long. Put your hands on the floor under your shoulders and press back, bringing your butt toward your heels without rolling your torso up. Instead, keep your chest on your thighs. You can bring your arms to either side of your legs and let your torso spread across your thighs, or reach your arms forward along the floor to stretch your back long. Hold this pose for five breath cycles.

Locust Variations

Come back down to your belly, with your arms over your head and your legs flat. Put your face gently against the floor. (If this bothers you, put a folded towel between your forehead and the floor.) On an inhale, lift your arms and legs slightly off the floor. Don't try to go high, just go to a place that's comfortable. When you exhale, don't drop your limbs completely back to the floor; instead, let them fall a little, and then inhale again, lifting your limbs a little higher. Do this for five breath cycles, and let your body flow with the breath rather than trying to force your body to hold the position. Come down to the start.

Knee Squeeze

Roll onto your back and lie in a neutral position, keeping your shoulders away from your ears and your body relaxed. On an inhale, bring your right knee in toward your chest and hold your knee with both hands. Take five breaths in this position, bringing your knee in closer to your chest each time you inhale. On an exhale go back to the start position. Repeat the same with your left knee, then with both knees. Relax back to the start position.

Supported Relaxation

Get some bed pillows. Lie on your back, and put one pillow under your knees, one under your lower back, and one under your neck and head. If you want, you can also place a pillow under each of your hands and lower arms. Close your eyes and breathe deeply. Hold this position for as long as you like. Don't be surprised if you fall asleep.

10-minute Full-body stretch

This stretch will work any time, anywhere. You can do it after a workout, when you wake up, before you go to bed, or after a long car ride. Some of the moves are yoga-based, while others are athletic stretches. One move flows into the next.

Star

Stand with your legs wide apart, abdominals contracted and shoulders down. Open your arms out wide to the side, being sure to keep your butt under your hips. Reach out wide with your arms and legs, pressing your feet into the floor and stretching your fingers wide. Drop your chin slightly so that the back of your neck is long. Hold this for 20 to 30 seconds while you breathe deeply.

Twist

Keeping your legs and arms wide, begin to turn to your right without letting your butt sway or your shoulders rise. Stay strong in your core and let your head follow your torso so that you're looking to the right. Continue to reach through your fingers and press down into your feet. Hold for 20 to 30 seconds. Come back to center and repeat to the left. Come back to center.

Side Stretch

Bring your legs together and bring your arms up over your head, shoulders away from your ears (in other words, don't hunch up). Contract your abs and start to stretch through your right side, reaching through your right arm and fingers toward the ceiling and being sure to keep both feet balanced on the floor. Lean a little to the left to feel the stretch in your right side. Keep breathing. Hold this for 20 to 30 seconds. Come back to the start position and go to the left.

Neck Stretch

Stand with your feet together and your arms by your sides, with your abs contracted and your shoulders down and back. Drop your head forward gently without forcing your chin to your neck, and hold for 20 to 30 seconds. Then, bring your chin toward your right shoulder. Hold this for

20 to 30 seconds. Come back to the center, and bring your chin to the left. Hold for 20 to 30 seconds. Bring your head back to its natural position, keeping your shoulders down. Widen your eyes and move your facial muscles around for a few seconds, stretching your mouth, too.

Now, keeping your shoulders down and your face relaxed, turn your head to the right gently, without forcing the stretch, and hold for 20 to 30 seconds. Come back to center and repeat to the left.

Chest and Upper Back Stretch

Keeping your shoulders down and your arms long, clasp your hands in front of your body, pushing your arms away from your torso as you pull away with your back. You should feel this in your upper back. Hold for 20 to 30 seconds. Now bring your arms long behind you (clasp your hands if you can). Keeping your shoulders down, push away from your torso to feel the stretch in your chest. Hold for 20-30 seconds.

Pelvis Stretch

Bring your hands to your lower back, fingers facing down. Contract your abs gently, with your feet hip width apart and your shoulders away from your ears. Gently push your pelvis forward.

Full Breath Meditation

Sit on the floor with crossed legs. Roll a bit back so that you're sitting fully on your sitting bones. Your back should be relaxed but long (don't slouch), and your chin should be slightly down so the back of your neck is long. Put your hands on your knees or in your lap.

Inhale through your nose and be conscious of your breath as you bring it into your head, then follow your breath as it drifts down your throat and into your shoulders, arms, chest, and belly. Follow the breath into your hips and legs, all the way down to your feet.

When you exhale, let the breath out slowly, feeling your body get a little smaller without the air filling it. Inhale again, filling your body up the same way you did the first time. Keep repeating this pattern, trying to make the breaths slower and deeper as you go on.

Be very conscious of your breath throughout the meditation, which should take about five minutes. If an anxious thought comes into your consciousness, just let it pass by, and if you become conscious that you've latched on to a thought, then consciously let it go and return to being conscious of your breath.

Early-morning Stretch

Start this stretch in bed, and then move onto the floor. Lying on your back with a flat pillow under your neck and head, tilt your chin down. Now, bring your right knee to your chest gently, and hold it with both hands for about 20 seconds. Repeat with the left leg. Tilt your head to the left and hold for 20 seconds, then tilt to the right. Stretch your arms out to the sides, reaching away from your torso for 20 seconds. Then bring your arms up over your head without scrunching up your shoulders.

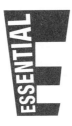

If you want, you can use this early-morning stretch time to remind yourself of your intentions or to offer a list of five things you're grateful for to help begin your day on a positive spiritual note, as well as a positive physical note. You might try reciting these things at the same time each day, joining them with your breath, almost like a ritual.

Sit up with your legs straight out in front of you, and gently clasp your hands in front of your chest, away from your body. Pull your arms away from your torso to stretch your back. Then reach your arms behind you, keeping your shoulders away from your ears, to stretch your chest.

Now, put your feet on the floor, and sit on the edge of your bed. Put your hands on your thighs or knees and bend from your waist to rest your upper body on your thighs. Let your head hang down, but do all of this gently, and don't try to force the stretch. Hold for 20 seconds. Unroll and stand up.

Inhale deeply and bring your arms up over your head, bending your knees. Then exhale, bringing your arms down and relaxing your knees. Do this three or four times.

Start your day!

At-the-office Stretch

This takes just a minute or two, but it will feel great. First, while sitting on a chair, put both feet on the floor, drop your shoulders away from your ears, and put your hands on your thighs. Take a few deep breaths, as slow as you can. Now, gently drop your head forward (don't force it) and hold for a few seconds. Now, roll your head to the right, chin toward your shoulder. Hold, roll your head back to center, and then roll your head to the left.

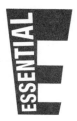

In a meeting? Tense? Bored? Without closing your eyes, start to focus on deepening the length of your inhales and exhales and, as you do this, focus on bringing your breath to each tense part of your body. This should relax you (on the exhale) and, at the same time, energize you (on the inhale).

Keeping your shoulders down, bring your arms in front of your chest, clasp your fingers, and reach your arms forward, stretching your back. Now stand up, put your hands on your lower back, and press your pelvis forward, leaning your upper body back. Bring your arms behind you and stretch your chest. If you can, bring one knee at a time up to your chest, then reverse that stretch and bring your heel to your butt, holding it with your hand. Go back to your day!

Chapter 11
Cross-training

People who cross-train have one main activity, such as running or yoga, but they complement this activity with other exercises. When done properly, cross-training gives the body everything it needs in terms of exercise and fitness. Elite athletes cross-train. For example, a football player's yoga practice makes him less vulnerable to injury when he plays on Sundays, a dancer's weight training makes her stronger for a performance, and a swimmer's walking helps her build bone. This chapter will give you an introduction to cross-training, as well as offer two programs you can try.

Picking a Main Sport or Activity

Most of us have one activity that we like and want to center our exercise schedules around. Picking this central exercise is helpful in cross-training because it gives our workouts a focus around which we can plan our other activities. The point of cross-training is to balance your activities so that you have cardio, strength, *and* mind-body/flexibility workouts in your schedule.

For example, let's say you want walking to be your main sport. In that case, you're not going to choose running as your other sport because that isn't really cross-training (since both are cardiovascular workouts). Instead, you'll want to find a way to incorporate strength training (maybe weight training or yoga), some flexibility (yoga or dancing, perhaps), and maybe some mind-body work (could also be yoga, or maybe meditation and Pilates) into your schedule.

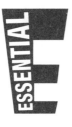

Picking a main activity doesn't mean you have to become an expert at that one thing, or that you even have to do it more often than you do your other activities. It is simply a way to organize your workout schedule so that you create a program that is properly balanced. Diversifying your activities helps you to enjoy the positive points of all the things you choose.

Of course, you can still do another cardio activity when you don't feel like walking. One or two swims a week along with your walks are obviously wonderful, but what you're looking for above all when you cross-train is a program that is balanced and makes your body stronger, leaner, and more refined, not a program that stresses your body in the same way during each workout.

Benefits of Different Activities

Every sport has its own set of benefits, as well as elements of fitness that it doesn't address or improve. Here are some sports and the ways they improve fitness.

	Aerobic	Weight Bearing	Muscular Strength/ Endurance	Flexibility	Caloric Expenditure
Swimming	Yes	No	Yes	Yes	Good
Biking	Yes	No	Lower and some upper	Some	Good
Running	Yes	Yes	Lower and some upper	Some	Best
Yoga	No	Yes	Yes	Yes	No
Weight training	Can be	Yes	Yes	No	Yes
Pilates	No	Yes	Yes	Yes	No
Kickboxing	Yes	Yes	Yes	A little	Yes

Of course, all activities accomplish more than one goal. When you take a walk, for example, you not only burn fat and make your heart stronger, but you also strengthen your leg, glute, and ab muscles, as well as build bone. So, it's fairly easy to pick three or four exercise types (such as yoga, running, and Pilates) and create a schedule that includes them all in an order that gives you the results you want.

Other Cross-training Benefits

Besides making your workout schedule interesting and fun, cross-training has other benefits. It gives you lots of options if the weather, your mood, or your schedule doesn't cooperate with your plans. You can even include group activities, which allows you to meet lots of different people.

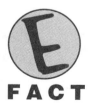

FACT

Cross-training increases the chance of weight loss by including both cardiovascular and strength-training work, which maximizes calorie burning both during the activity and over the course of a day. Also, cross-training will help you get better at each of your activities because the benefits of each carries over to every sport. Finally, cross-training helps prevent overuse injuries.

Another benefit is that you can rotate activities in and out of your schedule; for example, you can swim in the summer and take aerobics class in the winter. Likewise, you can adapt your routine over long periods of time, as you age, or as the seasons change.

Triathlon

The sport of triathlon is an interesting example of cross-training in action. In a triathlon, contestants take part in three activities, one after the other: swimming, biking, and running. Swimming is aerobic, improves your flexibility, uses most of the muscles in your body (improving muscular strength and endurance), and is not weight bearing (giving your skeletal system a rest from the pounding effect of running). Biking is aerobic, uses the hip and leg muscles as well as some of the upper body, works your balancing abilities, and, like swimming, is not weight bearing. Running is aerobic, uses the hip and leg muscles, and is weight bearing, but it is also jarring.

Even triathletes, who are extraordinarily fit, have to cross-train and do activities other than swimming, biking, and running. This occurs because, as you can see from the descriptions above, their sport (triathlon is considered one sport comprising three activities) doesn't include enough strength-training and flexibility. In fact, most triathletes make time for weightlifting and stretching, at the very least. This makes them better athletes and cuts down on their risk of injury.

Activity Choices

One way to create a cross-training schedule is to learn more about different activities, especially if you aren't actually interested in a particular sport. This is especially helpful if you like to take group exercise classes at the gym but don't know how to make sure you aren't doing too much of one type of exercise.

High-impact Aerobics

High-impact aerobics are usually weight-bearing (body weight and gravity are factors) activities that are repetitive in nature and cause varying degrees of jarring, jolting, or pounding to one's musculoskeletal system. Examples of such activities include running or jogging, walking, jumping rope.

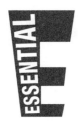

Having a certified instructor can weed out a lot of bad experiences, while at the same time, personality matters a lot. You want an instructor who is interested in you and your ability to follow along with the class. If you do not care for the instructor's choice of music, ask if that is the normal type of music in the class, and find another class if the music makes the hour intolerable.

You should monitor your heart rate in an aerobics class just as you do in other activities. Doing this keeps you aligned with your fitness goals. However, manually monitoring your heart rate in class when the music is loud is difficult, and prone to inaccuracy. In the time that you stop and search for your pulse, your heart rate has already dropped significantly from what it was during exercise. The best way to monitor your heart rate in an aerobics class is to wear your heart-rate monitor and check your intensity level while you are moving. Some classes may not challenge you enough; others might push you too hard. In either case, it is good to know your preferred heart rates during exercise so that you can maintain that rate or RPE during a class.

Low-impact Aerobics

Aerobic routines are dance-style movements that get you moving and shaking, and your heart a-poundin'. In low-impact aerobics, you move horizontally (up and back, side to side) a lot, but without absorbing much jarring and pounding. You usually have at least one foot on the ground, which rules out the high-impact activities like jumping and hopping. In high-impact aerobics routines, you experience more vertical movements like hopping and jumping, which naturally have a stronger impact on you when you land. Weight-bearing exercise is good for you, so you should not be too quick to assume that the "impact" part of high and low impact is a good or bad thing. It depends upon your fitness goals. There are also combination high/low classes. If those are not available, try alternating between the two styles. Classes vary by styles of movement as well as intensity of exercise and type of music.

Aside from low-impact aerobic routines, there are other low-impact aerobic activities that are non-weight-bearing and that generate little, if any, jarring, jolting, or pounding to one's musculoskeletal system. Such activities include swimming, water aerobics, bicycling, rowing, cross-country skiing, stairclimbing, and using elliptical machines.

If you like dance, doing aerobics routines is great. If you have rhythm, coordination, and the ability to follow or remember dance-style movements, you will catch on quickly and have a great aerobic workout. However, if this is your first-ever dance class, or if you opted for tennis and skipped dance at summer camp, you could be in for a tough time.

In-line Skating

This outdoor fitness activity is often better known as in-line skating, or roller blading from the brand name Roller Blade. Since the debut of Roller Blades in 1980, other manufacturers have also been producing these ice skates on wheels. I call them that because an in-line skate closely resembles an alpine ski boot, and the four-in-a-row wheel alignment resembles a wheeled ice skate.

In-line skating can be aerobic; it works the gluteal (rear end) muscles; and it refreshes the areas of the brain responsible for balance and coordination. It can also humble even the experienced skater with a single fall. Adults typically work hard to master in-line skating; kids seem to pick it up quickly and keep on going without missing a beat. Learning in-line skating is great for your sense of humor as long as you are able to laugh at yourself.

How to In-line Skate

The skating motion involves alternating your legs, pushing sideways against the ground, and then gliding. This movement works the very large and powerful lateral muscles of the hips and buttocks, so it is easy to gain speed quickly. Gliding swiftly over the pavement on your feet is fun. But until you have mastered slowing and stopping, the fun can come to an unplanned and abrupt halt. So if you are mentally ready for the experience, be prepared with the right equipment, and practice your stopping and slowing skills. You can consider yourself an experienced skater when you can control your skates and stop at will.

In-line Skating Necessities

Whenever the ground is clear and dry, you can skate. If it is snowing, change over to your ice skates and hit the rink. In the fall months, watch for fallen leaves and debris, both of which can interrupt a nice glide.

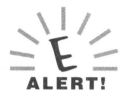

In-line skating is free, since you can skate around a park or on the sidewalk. However, there are some costs related to equipment. In-line skates cost approximately $75 to $150, depending on quality. A helmet is around $35, and you should also wear wrist, elbow, and knee guards, which are about $20 for a set.

Your skates (really, the boots on the skates) should fit snugly so that your feet do not move around inside them. This gives you better control when you are skating. The boot (or bootie) usually has a foam interior covered in hard-shell plastic, which gives you some ventilation and comfort. However, if you have weak ankles, this may not be the sport for you. Or maybe it could be—you will surely build ankle strength if you can stay with it long enough.

Cardio Machines

One of the best ways to cross-train is to use a different cardio machine each time you go to the gym. Unless you're on a specific type of program, such as walking or bicycling, then changing machines is a great way to work your heart, burn calories, and keep yourself interested in your cardio training. More variety means less boredom!

In terms of calorie burning and heart-pumping effectiveness, the elliptical trainer is your best bet. It is low-impact, but it allows you to burn more calories and work your heart harder than a walk would, be it on the road or on a treadmill. Most people find the elliptical trainer fun and easier to use, and they don't feel the intensity of their workout as much as they do on other machines, especially rowers and stationary cycles.

Most personal trainers will also tell you that another great machine is the rower, which works all of your body efficiently and strengthens the heart. Unfortunately, most people can actually feel how hard the rower makes you work, unlike with the elliptical trainer, which allows you to work hard but not feel your effort as intensely.

You can switch machines during one workout, or alternate machines each time you head to a gym. For example, here are two sample cardio cross-training exercise sessions:

- **5-minute warm-up:** Start the treadmill at 3.0 mph and go up to 3.5 mph.
- **20-minute interval program:** Use the elliptical trainer at an RPE between 5 and 8.
- **5-minute steady state:** Use the rower at an RPE of 6.
- **10-minute cooldown:** Use the stationary cycle, going down to an RPE of 2-3.
- **5-minute warm-up:** Stationary cycle at an RPE of 2-5.
- **5-minute steady state:** Use the stationary cycle at an RPE of 6.
- **15-minute hill-climbing program:** Use the treadmill with the ramp going up at an RPE between 6 and 8.
- **10-minute steady state:** Use the elliptical trainer at an RPE of 6.
- **5-minute cooldown:** Use the treadmill, going down to a slow walk.

Don't worry about looking funny moving from machine to machine. Real gym rats practice cross-training programs more than they stick to one machine over time. It's much more effective to challenge your body with variety.

Don't Overdo It!

Injuries and fatigue are, unfortunately, part of staying in shape, although of course, injury and fatigue are also part of being deconditioned and out of shape. The difference is the type of injury, the reason for the fatigue, and the way you handle both.

Exercising a lot is great, but exercising too much is dangerous. For one thing, your body needs rest as much as it needs activity. In other words, everything in moderation. Even professional athletes balance their intense workout programs with lots of rest because they have exerted themselves so much.

This is not to say you have to spend entire days sleeping or being inactive. It simply means that training—intense exercise with a goal—cannot be done seven days a week.

For example, you can take a walk every day, but you can't take an interval walk every day. You can swim every day, but some of those swims should be fun, not timed laps. If you do yoga every day, some of your poses should be restorative.

If you feel very tired, listen to your body and don't push yourself through a workout. Instead, give yourself a day of rest and understand that you will work out on the following day. Don't be afraid that you will stop exercising forever. The reality is that ignoring signs of overuse and overtraining tend to lead to stopping exercise, but appropriate rest will help you stay in shape and keep you motivated.

It's okay to exercise if you have a little cold, but anything more than that and you're overheating and overtaxing your body enough to make it difficult for your body to fight the infection or bug that is invading your system.

Cold symptoms include no fever or a very low one (99 to 100 degrees Fahrenheit), no body ache or a slight one, mild fatigue, and congested nose and sneezing. A cold comes on slowly, and having a headache with a cold is rare.

Flu symptoms are a high fever that can last three to four days, headache, body aches, and exhaustion (which can last up to a few weeks). The flu comes on suddenly, and congestion and sneezing are rare. You should never exercise when you have the flu, and, in fact, you should wait a few days and ramp up your routine slowly even after you're all better.

Making a Schedule

As you've learned, it's best to pick a main activity that you will make the center of your workout schedule. Most people create a weekly workout schedule, so get out your calendar.

Let's say you take three walks a week with a friend in your neighborhood and you know that those walks provide good cardio training. You realize that you need to add some strength training, so you decide to buy some dumbbells and an exercise DVD to use in your home twice a week. Now you want to add a little flexibility to your program, but you're running out of time between your job and your family. You decide that, in this case, all you can manage is some stretching in front of the TV in the evenings.

That's fine, by the way. Cross-training doesn't have to be intense. However, you might want to invest in a stretching DVD (they are usually fairly short) to give you some ideas on what to do.

However, let's say you are someone who likes a lot of different activities, such as walking, swimming, weight training, yoga, and Pilates. How can you fit them all in? Chances are, you can't, not in one week anyway. If that's the case, think about the benefits and time costs of each activity, and try to be sure you are doing two different types of activities on consecutive days. For example, don't swim on Monday, dance on Tuesday, and walk on Wednesday. Stick some weight training in between all of those cardio activities.

Two Effective Cross-training Programs

The first cross-training program that follows is centered around the treadmill, but you could substitute any cardio machine for those sessions. The strength workouts can be done on machines or with free weights. Or, you could do a strength/flexibility activity, such as yoga and Pilates, on those days. The bonus workouts are actually fun activities and aren't really workouts with programs, but are instead just good fitness-oriented things to do.

Cross-training Program #1

Monday: 40-minutes using the hill climbing program on a treadmill

Tuesday: 25-minute strength training

Wednesday: 40 minute interval session on a treadmill

Thursday: 25-minute strength training

Friday: 40 minute interval session on a treadmill

Saturday: Long hike

Sunday: Swim

Cross-training Program #2

This program is centered around a race—the triathlon. This person wants to compete for the first time and so has to fit biking, swimming, and running into her schedule, but she also needs to strength-train and stretch for optimum fitness. The following would be a one-week program in a twelve-week training schedule. Because she's working out so intensely, she needs to truly rest on her days off.

Monday: 45-minute bike ride, 15-minute Pilates-based strength and stretch program

Tuesday: 30-minute swim

Wednesday: 30-minute run, 15-minute Pilates-based strength and stretch program

Thursday: Rest

Friday: 30-minute swim

Saturday: 20-minute swim, 20-minute bike ride, 30-minute run

Sunday: Rest

Chapter 12
Gyms

Perhaps the world is made up of two types of people: those who love gyms—the variety of classes, the camaraderie of working out with other people, and the choice between classes and all of the equipment—and those people who would sooner stick a fork in their eye than let other people see them exercise. Whichever group you fall into, here's where you'll find out more about how to choose the best gym or why, surprisingly, a gym membership would work for you, no matter what type of person you are now.

Are You a Gym Person?

Before you find out about gyms, you actually need to know a few things about yourself to see whether you're someone who needs a gym. Will you be inspired by working out in public, or embarrassed? Don't try to become something you're not. If you're not someone who wants to change in a locker room, sweat in public, use the same weights as strangers, and have to follow gym etiquette (smiling at strangers, using machines for allotted time periods, and wiping everything down), then maybe a gym is not for you. Don't kid yourself; gyms aren't perfect, and they aren't the only way to get into shape. So if your first reaction to a gym is "ick," then skip this chapter and read further on in this book for other ways to create an exercise program.

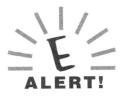

ALERT!

Are you going to use the gym enough to make its price worthwhile? Let's say a gym membership is $750 per year, or $62.50 per month. If you go twice a week, or about eight times a month, then each visit costs you over $7, which is pretty expensive. On the other hand, if the gym is conveniently located and you go four or five times a week, then each visit costs just a few dollars a month, and that is pretty cost efficient.

Is there an activity or piece of equipment—such as a pool—that you can't get anyplace else? If you love to swim but don't have a pool in your backyard—and if swimming is really the only way you enjoy exercise—then spend the money to join a gym or club that has the pool you will most enjoy. If there is an activity—whether it's horseback riding or swimming, yoga or dance—you really want to do, then don't force yourself to create an exercise program without the activity you love. Instead, start with what you love, and the fitness will follow.

There are practical reasons to join a gym, though, no matter what kind of person you are. First, there is always someone around to watch you perform an exercise and make sure you're doing it right. Also, there are lots of machines and choices for workouts, as well as lots of options for classes and activities. Usually gyms make an effort to bring in new equipment regularly, which makes your workouts safer and more fun.

You can make friends and use group support to help you with your commitment to exercise. Also, gyms often have nutritionists and other people on staff who can help you reach your goals. Gyms allow you to try things you wouldn't normally try because they constantly change and update classes.

Finally, even if the money seems like a problem, sometimes it can be an incentive for you. In other words, if you're spending money on membership fees, you will be inspired to go to the gym regularly. Likewise, sometimes a gym membership helps to motivate people. They have somewhere different to go that's reserved just for exercise—it's something to look forward to and plan for.

Differences Between Gyms

Gyms range from inexpensive, usually around $40 a month, to wildly expensive, tens of thousands of dollars each year. The price usually reflects a number of things: location, number of members (the more expensive a club, the more exclusive it is), the age of the equipment, the number of trainers, the education level of the trainers, and cleanliness. Expensive gyms also offer their clients towels and high-quality workout clothes, as well as toiletries.

But most gyms fall within a moderate price range, depending on where you live, i.e., if you live in an expensive city or suburb, the average gym cost will be slightly more than it is in a more downscale neighborhood. Whatever its price, though, everyone needs to look at a few things about a gym—plus know a few things about themselves—before they make a commitment (and sometimes, it is a commitment) to join a gym.

Cost

Don't join a gym that you can't afford or that forces you to make a long-term financial commitment if you really aren't sure you are going to go. Gym staffs—and regular gym members—scoff at the people who sign up around the New Year (resolution time) only to disappear in February. Gyms get rich off those people because they continue to pay monthly dues even if they only attend regularly in the month of January. In fact, most gyms wouldn't be able to actually hold—much less offer equipment and training to—all of their members if they all actually showed up. Gyms actually count on members paying but not attending.

Cleanliness

Of equal importance, though, is cleanliness. Nothing is more disgusting—or more dangerous to your health—than a dirty gym. Sweat, hair in drains, fungi in locker rooms—they're not just gross; these things can truly compromise your health. So, if you walk through a gym, look carefully at the equipment, the bathrooms, and the people using the equipment (are they carrying towels, do they seem clean?) because you don't want to give your money to a gym that isn't sparkling.

Daycare

Some moms love gyms because the gym gives them a chance to get out of the house and be active, while also providing a little baby-sitting and child care. This child care, however, can range from excellent to dangerous. Don't just let your kids stay somewhere without finding out more about the child care director and her staff. Does the director have a degree or equivalent experience in taking care of children (specifically kids the same age as yours?), and is the child care facility stocked with clean toys and activities? What are the rules and regulations about snacks (particularly if your child has a food allergy)? Visit the child care center a couple of times and notice what the staff is doing. Are they sitting around looking bored? Are they interacting with the children and entertaining them? This can be an expensive added-on cost to your gym membership, and you should make sure you're getting what you pay for.

Activities and Equipment

Does the gym specialize in certain activity or classes, and how is the equipment room? Is there enough equipment available during the times you'll be there? Not everyone needs the most up-to-date machinery, but there should be enough equipment to ensure that you will get to do what you want when you arrive at the gym's door. Look around when you go for a gym tour; if there isn't one free machine, then chances are you won't get to do what you want when you join.

Using Machines

Now, let's get to the weight machines. One of the selling factors of most gyms, including places such as Curves, is that they feature circuit strength machines. A circuit, as mentioned previously, is a trail or path around the strength machines. So, basically, you will go into the gym and use one machine at a time—someone at the gym will actually show you how to use each machine and explain (one hopes) which muscle each machine works.

Typically each machine isolates one muscle, so the rest of your body is technically at rest—sitting, usually—and the machine allows you to simply move one muscle or muscle group, which allows you to use a heavier weight. If you, for example, do a bicep curl with a dumbbell, you'll probably use five or eight pounds, but if you use a Nautilus machine (that's a brand name) you might be able to lift twice that.

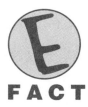

FACT

The most important thing you should do and know about weight machines versus free weights is that the only thing that truly matters—truly—is your preference. There is no one right way to create a strength-training program, except, of course, to be safe, and we'll cover that in a minute.

Weight machines, like anything else, have pros and cons. First, they are quite effective—just as effective as free weights and bands. Second, they are actually very easy to use. Third, because the whole sequence is done in the order the machines are in, you don't have to think that much about what you have to do. Just follow the path—or circuit—and you're good to go.

The negatives to weight machines are few. First, if you aren't of average height, the machines might not be for you. They are designed to fit the "average male," so if you're shorter than 5'8" (or much taller, for that matter) then you might feel uncomfortable or even not be able to do the exercises because your body won't line up with the machine properly.

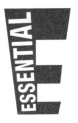

You may find it boring to just move from one machine to the next. Some people like putting a little thought into their workout, and not everyone enjoys isolating one muscle at a time. It's much more engaging to have to use your whole body during any given exercise, even just a bicep curl, than to sit down and move only your forearms.

People who enjoy strength-training—and there are many men and women who swear by it—tend to mix up their routines, using free weights for some exercises, bands for others, and machines for others, based on how much weight they want to lift and how comfortable they are with any give exercise.

Paying for a Gym Membership

This is just a brief word about something you might know, and that is that many health insurance plans pay for—at least partially—gym memberships (as well as some weight-loss programs). So, if you have health insurance, be sure to call and find out. And before you join a gym, call your health insurance company to find out what gyms belong to their reimbursement program, because that might help you decide which one you should join.

There are a number of ways to help motivate yourself to go the gym. As you read, you should think of your payments to the gym as being cheaper per visit if you go a lot, but especially expensive if you never go. But here are some other ideas:

- Join with a friend, and commit to carpooling there and giving each other pep talks and rewards to support each other.
- Sign up with a trainer for a session a month. Even though this is even more money, the trainer will get you on a program and update it each month so that you will be assured of making progress and will have someone who will regularly check in on you. If the trainer tries to make

you buy more sessions, find a new trainer (unless you think she's on the up-and-up and you do, in fact, need more help and coaching).

- Pay yourself to go. If your health plan does include reimbursement of your gym costs, you probably will have to prove that you're using the gym. Promise yourself that you will use that money as a reward, not as repayment for the gym's costs, but as a special trip to the theater, a new piece of furniture, or a piece of jewelry. Or, best of all, new clothes for your new body!

- Create a contest. How many new classes can you try in a month? How many minutes can you add to your elliptical workout? How much more weight can you lose in eight visits? Aim for progress, but in a fun way.

Remember the concept of active intentions from Chapter 2. Instead of saying you will lose weight, list the two classes you will attend each week. Instead of saying you will fit into your old jeans, write down that you will go to the gym three times a week. In other words, include the gym in your plan, schedule, and intentions.

Two Gym Programs

As mentioned previously, many gyms, such as Curves, have their own programs, and they will put you on their machines and explain how to use their equipment. Don't dismiss these programs, either. If you haven't been working out for a while or if you feel uncomfortable around gym equipment, these programs will work.

Most often, though, if you join a gym, they will give you one or two training sessions with their personal trainers. And that trainer will put you on a program using the machines and equipment the gym has. Most gyms have the equipment in the two following programs. There are two ways to go to the gym. First, you can go five or six days a week and alternate the days you do cardio work and the days you do strength work. For example:

Monday:	40 minutes on the elliptical trainer
Tuesday:	Full-body strength-training program

Wednesday: 40 minutes on the treadmill

Thursday: Full-body strength-training program

Friday: 40 minutes on the elliptical trainer

Or you can take classes at your gym, although, of course, once again, you need to mix it up to be sure your week includes all the elements of a well-rounded fitness program. For example:

Monday: 50-minute step class

Tuesday: 1-hour-and-15-minute strength-training class

Wednesday: 90-minute yoga class

Thursday: 50-minute step class

Friday: 1-hour-and-15-minute strength-training class

Saturday: Swim

Another option is to head to the gym three times a week and combine your cardio and strength training each time you work out. As you will see, these programs take less time, but they can be just as effective. The trick is to make the workouts more intense. For example:

Monday: 20-minute interval program on the elliptical trainer, 20-minute full-body strength-training routine

Wednesday: 20-minute interval program on the treadmill, 20-minute full-body strength-training routine

Friday: 20-minute interval program on the elliptical trainer, 20-minute full-body strength-training routine

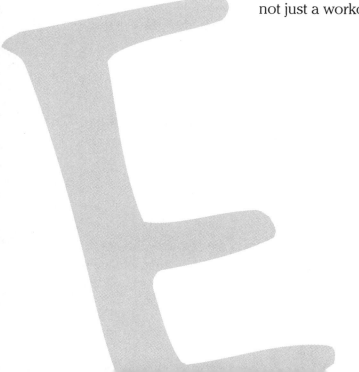

Chapter 13
Lifestyle Changes

Life in the twenty-first century is centered around sitting: sitting in the car, sitting at work, and sitting when we relax. The result? Weight gain and loss of muscle tone and shape. In order to get fit, you need to create a life that is active, not just a workout program.

The Modern Problem

Think about the physical activity that has been lost through the following modern conveniences. We drive instead of walk. We use e-mail instead of going to the post office. We use a food processor instead of mixing dough. We watch television instead of walking to the movies. We call people instead of walking over to their houses. We have food delivered rather than going out to eat. We use leaf blowers, riding lawn mowers, and power tools. We use escalators instead of stairs.

Because we have reduced the time we spend doing even simple activities that used more of our arms, legs, back, heart, and lungs, our bodies have become weaker and less capable of work. This rise in inactivity has been devastating to our health. Truly, we have witnessed the meaning of the "use it or lose it" phenomenon. When we don't use our bodies, we lose the ability to use them.

This grim reality is described by Dr. Kenneth Cooper in his revolutionary book *Aerobics*: "A body that isn't used deteriorates. The lungs become inefficient, the heart grows weaker, the blood vessels less pliable, the muscles lose tone and the body generally weakens throughout, leaving it vulnerable for a whole catalog of illness and disease. Your whole system for delivering oxygen almost literally shrivels up." The bottom line is this: We are meant to be active, and our health depends upon it. When the body is used, it thrives; when it isn't, it merely survives.

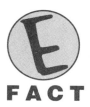

FACT

Americans watch an average of more than four hours of TV a day, or two full months of TV a year. According to Dr. William Dietz, Director of the Division of Nutrition and Physical Activity at the Centers for Disease Control, "The easiest way to reduce inactivity is to turn off the TV set. Almost anything else uses more energy than watching TV."

In 1900, the leading causes of deaths in the United States were not at all related to lifestyle, but were instead diseases and infections that science had not yet figured out. They included pneumonia, tuberculosis, gastroenteritis, and influenza. Since then medicine has found the solutions to those problems, but our lifestyle has created new ones. The leading causes of death in 1990 were heart disease, stroke, cancer, and accidents.

As you can see, the leading causes of death in 1900 were biological in nature and could be reduced through vaccines and treatments. The leading causes of death in 1990, on the other hand, were related to lifestyle and could be reduced through fitness. Fitness as prevention is effective, simple, and inexpensive compared to the cost of the medical treatment for those diseases.

Getting Back to Basics

While you may be happy that you don't have to garden, clean your house, or live the life of your parents and grandparents, your body is not that happy about it. In fact, your body would be thrilled if you could live in the 1950s. Oh sure, no one wants you to be stuck cleaning and cooking all day, but a little bit of activity during the day would be the perfect way to stay in shape.

You might be surprised to learn that housewives in the 1950s burned over 1,000 calories more per day and consumed 1,000 calories less than women of today do, even though today's woman is certainly busier with a wider variety of activities. Fifty years ago, women spent three hours a day doing household chores, and walked an hour a day to do their shopping. They also ate healthier meals, with more vegetables, and had fewer snacks. In fact, the numbers reveal the truth: Women today eat an average of 2,178 calories a day, but only burn off 556 through daily activities. In 1952, the average woman ate 1,818 calories a day and burned 1,512 calories.

Now, does this mean you should give up your washing machine and dryer, your dishwasher, and your vacuum cleaner? Of course not. But it does serve as proof that our lifestyles have created the weight and health problems facing us today. Knowing that should inspire you to rearrange your life so that you get more activity. In truth, movement will help our bodies, not being sedentary.

Gardening

Years ago, only wealthy people employed gardeners and landscapers, but today gardeners and landscapers work for everyone in the neighborhood, even in middle-class neighborhoods. And what are the owners—and kids—in these middle-class home doing while someone else is raking their leaves? Often, watching TV, eating, or surfing the Internet.

And that's a shame, because digging, raking, and planting are moderate-intensity activities, equivalent to taking a brisk walk. Even better? Tough gardening chores such as mowing the lawn with a push mower, chopping wood, and shoveling are comparable to skiing or playing doubles tennis. These activities do not replace true exercise routines, but they are a perfect way to reverse the curse of inactivity.

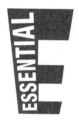

To make gardening safer, remember that when you're weeding or planting, bend at the knees rather than at the waist. Also, try to alternate your grip when using tools. Additionally, don't do too much. You shouldn't work longer in your garden than you would take a walk, for example. Finally, stretch when you need to and don't sit in one position for too long.

Gardening offers one more important benefit, though. It is psychologically uplifting. Being outside, growing food or flowers, interacting with nature, possibly working with other members of your family, and (sometimes literally) seeing the fruits of your labors are rewarding in ways other activities aren't. Of course, as with your other workouts, make sure you schedule your gardening and write it down in your calendar.

Housecleaning

Now, this is a funny thing. These days, many people think of housecleaning as beneath them, even though they are proud of their clean homes. In other words, as with gardening, they let someone else do the work.

And that's a shame, because housecleaning is, in many ways, the perfect cross-training workout. It combines cardio (especially if you're scrubbing bathrooms or floors), resistance training in your upper body, and flexibility (because you are moving around a lot and constantly changing position). In many ways, housecleaning is like dancing—it's constant motion. And cleaning your house yourself will save you money!

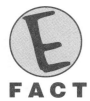

FACT

The following are the activities that can make a change in your body, including your heart and muscles: vacuuming, dusting, washing floors, scrubbing bathrooms, and washing windows. Because of differences in body size, activities, and energy output, no one knows exactly how many calories you'll burn, but rough estimates are anywhere from 100 to 300 calories per hour, depending on your intensity level.

Another very effective strategy is to clean your house in 10-minute, 20-minute, or 30-minute breaks in the evening, especially if the TV is usually on. Get up during commercials and wash your sinks, or turn off the TV during that half-hour show you don't really like and do the whole bathroom. Not only will you burn a nice number of calories, but the energy blast will lighten your mood and you'll be happy with the reward of a cleaner house!

Dancing

Even if you have two left feet, turn on your CD player or put the iPod in its docking station, and start moving. Whether it's in your bedroom or your living room or a local club or studio, dancing is wonderful exercise.

In fact, aerobics as a form of exercise got started as dance, an offshoot of jazz dance (sort of like what the Rockettes do). Because you move quickly (even ballroom dancers dance relatively fast) and use all of your limbs, you burn a ton of calories dancing. The funny thing about dancing, too, is that all you really need is a sense of rhythm and an enjoyment of music—you can be good at it no matter what your size or shape.

Taking a dance class, whether it's ballet, belly-dancing, or swing dancing, can get you into shape and is a great way to be social. But you can also dance by yourself in your home with just the radio on.

Here's a list of different dance styles, their benefits, and their calorie-burning count for a moderate intensity for 30 minutes (keep in mind that most dance classes are at least 60 minutes):

- **Ballroom dancing:** Burns 150 calories an hour. Strengthens leg, shoulder, ab, arm, back, and glute muscles; increases flexibility. Improves concentration. Only increases heart strength if you do fast steps, such as swing dancing.
- **Salsa dancing:** Burns 170 calories an hour. Strengthens leg, shoulder, ab, arm, back, and glute muscles. Also increases flexibility. Strengthens the heart.
- **Ballet:** Burns 150 calories per hour. Strengthens leg, shoulder, ab, arm, back, and glute muscles. Also increases flexibility. You need concentration and stamina. Does not increase cardio power.
- **Country line dancing:** Burns 125 calories an hour. Strengthens leg, shoulder, ab, arm, back, and glute muscles.
- **Disco dancing:** Burns 175 calories an hour. Strengthens leg, shoulder, ab, arm, back, and glute muscles. Strengthens the heart.

Running Errands

When it seems as if you're about to have a busy day, you get into your car with a long list of errands you need to run. Here's an idea: put a step counter on your hip to actually see how many steps you are taking when you run errands. It's probably fewer than you think. Unfortunately.

The truth is, when we "run" errands, we are really just sitting in our cars between very short bouts of walking into stores and then quickly walking out. Think about it. You take twenty steps out to your car (and this is being generous), get in, and ride probably less than a mile to your dry cleaner, for example. You get out of the car and walk twenty steps to the counter. You stand for a few minutes, get your clothes, walk the twenty steps back to your car, and then drive to your next errand. Although this might have taken 10 minutes, you really didn't move very much.

To fix this problem, use your errand time as a source of exercise. If you can, walk from errand to errand. If that's impossible because you live in the suburbs, no one walks, and there are no sidewalks, then try to group your errands together so that your errands for one day are in the same general area and you don't have to keep getting in and out of your car. That alone might save you a half-hour. Now, use that half-hour for exercise. You could do an exercise video, take a walk in the park, or go for a swim. Each of those activities would be more beneficial to your body (not to mention the environment) than running errands.

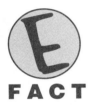

FACT

If you run five different errands to five different locations, you will have spent an hour taking about 100 steps, which is not much better than sitting on your couch. One of the reasons errands are tiring is because they are boring.

This statistic surprised experts and lay people alike: Adults and children are significantly less active on weekends than they are during the week. The image of people playing football outside or taking walks is a nice one, but it's an illusion. The truth is, most people sit on their couches, sleep later, watch more movies, and, most significantly, spend more time in their cars on the weekend.

Therefore, here are a few things you can do to create an active weekend:

- Once again, turn to your calendar to schedule your time. But on weekends, not only should you schedule your workouts, but also you should schedule some fun. Hikes, ice skating, a day at the beach, a bike ride with the whole family—all of these activities will keep you out of the house and moving your body.
- Don't drive on Sunday, and turn off the TV. If you can, spend time at your house, being busy. Wash your car, garden, play a game of

touch football. But again, don't turn on the TV, because that actually burns fewer calories than sitting in your car.

- Indulge yourself without food. Don't skip the fun, of course (even if that does mean dinner out), but try to find ways to enjoy yourself without eating too much, or non-nutritiously.

Community Activism

In many towns, children can't walk to school anymore, but must be bused or driven. It's difficult to find places to walk and play, and many children have physical education in school only once a week—if that.

Here are five qualities active towns share:

- Safe places to walk
- An inexpensive gym, often a YMCA
- Bike trails and bike awareness
- Support for your favorite activities—whether it's a place to swim, a yoga studio, or a fun place to dance
- Health and physical education classes in schools, as well as recess

Active people often seek out active places to live. They head to Boulder, Colorado, for the skiing, or Honolulu for the surfing. As for the rest of us, we live where we live, and we need to find ways to help turn our car-obsessed, fitness-discouraging towns into active places to live. Following are some ideas on how to help your town become more active.

Get Sidewalks Built

Many states and townships have matching programs that help communities get sidewalks built. If you and your neighbors want sidewalks in your area (and you should; they have been shown to increase the amount of walking people do), first go to a town meeting to find out if there is money in the budget for this, and to see what steps you need to take to have the sidewalks built. If someone tells you it's not possible to have the sidewalk built, enlist the help of your assemblyman or town council person to see where there might be budget money. Ask for support from both the community and the officials, and don't stop when you hear the word "no." No is only a step in the process, it is not the final answer.

Encourage a Gym to Come to Town

Curves, Bally, the YMCA—there are numerous gym chains and companies that are always looking for communities to serve where they can earn a profit. Attend a town Chamber of Commerce meeting and find out if an exercise organization has ever expressed an interest in your town. If you attend a gym or Y in a nearby community, see if you can speak to the CEO or president of that location, and express your idea to them. Or ask a local university if it would offer evening exercise classes at the local high school.

Create Bike Trails and Bike Awareness

If there is unused natural space in your community, consider contacting a group such as Rails to Trails (see Appendix A) or other public fitness organizations, because community fitness trails have been shown to increase activity levels, especially in previously sedentary and lower-income populations. In fact, a Saint Louis University School of Public Health study of communities in southeastern Missouri, where walking trails had recently been built, found that nearly 40 percent of people with access had used the trails, and that more than 55 percent of trail walkers had increased the amount of walking they did since they began using the trails. The Saint Louis University researchers also found that women were more than twice as likely as men to report that they had increased the amount of walking they did since they had begun to use the walking trails.

Get Support for Your Favorite Activities

Whether it's a place to swim, a yoga studio, or a fun place to dance, the best way to support this type of program is to go to a school and find a teacher, then work with him or her to find a location. Yoga studios host martial arts and dance classes, while public schools will allow adults to take all types of classes at night. If it's a pool you're looking for, you might have to go the local government route and find a way to get the community behind a common goal.

Encourage Physical Education Classes and Recess

Recess has become a hot topic for local school boards and parent-teacher organizations because with budget cuts, many schools no longer have the resources to pay people to watch kids while they play. At the same time, more demanding scholastic expectations have convinced many parents that recess is a waste of time. But it isn't. In the first place, sitting all day is as detrimental to your children as it is to you, both to their physical health and their intellectual health. There are numerous organizations that support this idea, including government agencies, so go before your school board and fight for this important time in your child's day. See Appendix A for resources.

New Ways to Relax

Changing the way you live your life takes a lot of energy and commitment. And unfortunately, you probably reward yourself with leisure and food. For example, you might relax by sitting in front of the TV with a bowl of ice cream. But this reward will counteract all of the improvements you've made in your life. TV and food are a deadly combination—literally—when it comes to your health, your fitness, and your weight.

So, when it comes time for you to relax and reward yourself, consider these ideas:

- A manicure and pedicure
- Sparkling water and grapes at the movies (sneak them in!)
- A new book or a CD
- Downloading some music to walk or dance to
- Taking a walk with a friend
- Going to a museum
- Experimenting with a new healthy recipe
- Working on a craft project

Remember that almost any activity, even a sedentary one, is better for your body than TV and mindless eating.

Chapter 14

Easy Fitness for the Office

Contrary to popular belief, chairs are actually pretty tough on the body. You might think that because they "give you a rest" they are helping your body relax, but chairs actually present two problems. First, the position they force your body into shortens some muscles (those in the front of the body) and lengthens others (those in the back of the body), which creates an imbalance in the body, leading to pain and injury. It's time to make your eight (or more) hours in the office (not to mention your commute) more active.

14

The Problem with Modern Work

Like the increased time we spend in cars and in front of the TV, most of us work more hours than our parents and grandparents did. And while we certainly have more money and live at a higher standard than our parents and grandparents, we have paid a price for the money we earn.

For one thing, while we do, as you have read, enjoy healthier bodies—fewer deaths from infectious illnesses, for example, our quality of life has changed. We are stressed, we are fatter, and we have sacrificed time with our families and friends.

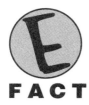

FACT

By the time a child leaves high school, she will have sat for more than 40,000 hours, over half of her waking life. This is one reason it is so important to encourage your child to be active when she's not in school, and, also to make sure your child's school gives her time to be as active as possible during the day. Too much sitting as she grows up will hurt her body when she's older.

Although it would be wonderful to start a fitness revolution, it is more realistic, at least in this moment, to instead be aware of this situation. Accept that your life is not as active as it should be, and that much of the reason for that is your job. Therefore, one important thing you can do is change the way you live during your work day.

Sitting Differently

Sitting too much and sitting improperly are equally troublesome to your body, but we're going to tackle sitting improperly first. Consider the human body, which was designed to move, and, at the very least, stand or squat. Chairs and couches were not part of the package until Man decided he could invent a better, more comfortable way for us to sit.

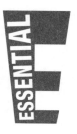

Sitting doesn't hurt while we're doing it because we're not holding up our own weight. So, while we might feel uncomfortable twinges in our hips or lower backs while we sit, our bodies don't tend to hurt because they don't get tired. But that doesn't mean sitting doesn't hurt us. We just feel the pain later when we try to move as we were meant to.

There's only one problem: while we are comfortable in chairs and couches, because we rest in them, our bodies aren't really that happy. First, sitting crunches up our hip flexors (the muscles that run from our lower ribs to our hips) while, at the same time, stretching our lower back and butt muscles. And we stay in this position for hours at a time.

Imagine if you were to stay in a lunge or a squat or the top of a pushup for hours. It would hurt, right? And you would change positions, right?

We also slouch when we sit, sinking into chairs and allowing our core muscles to not work, so that when we do need to stand or walk or do anything active, our muscles are too weak to accomplish our goals efficiently. Following are some suggestions to counteract these problems.

Try Standing Up

Many companies will construct work areas at which you can stand. While the idea may seem tiring to you at first, after a day or two, you'll really notice the difference in the way your back feels. Want to know a secret? This entire book—all 85,000 words—was written standing up. My back felt (and still feels) great.

Get a Ball

Another thing people are trying is sitting on their exercise balls at their desks. This is a good idea because it forces you to use your core muscles as you sit. One problem, though, is that it can be tiring, because you are, in fact, exercising while you work, so have a chair (or a place to stand) nearby during your workday.

Make Your Workstation Inconvenient

If you have to stand up to reach for your stapler, bend over to get your tape dispenser, and move across your office or cubicle to grab a file, you'll unconsciously move more, which will counteract the problems of sitting too much.

"Active" Jobs

Few of us have truly "active" jobs—ones in which our bodies work in all different ways equally throughout the day, ones in which we have adequate amounts of rest, ones in which we work in balance. Instead, even those people who are fortunate enough not to sit all day, are also very often, forced to ask their bodies to perform in an imbalanced manner—hammering with their right hand, standing hunched over an assembly line, or needing to lift and support people heavier than themselves under stressful conditions.

How to Really Be in an Active Job

There are a few things you can do if you have what is traditionally considered an "active" job. First, get honest about the reality of what you are asking your body to do. Instead of trying to convince yourself, for example, that your job is enough to keep you fit and healthy, recognize that you require an exercise program that does two things. First, it should keep you fit and healthy enough to do your job, and second, it should balance out any out-of-balance activity you have to do on a day-to-day basis.

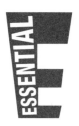

Nurses walk all day and help support patients in and out of beds. Construction workers climb and lift and favor work with one arm and hold one position for long amounts of time. Factory workers stand and do repetitive motions for hours at a time. These are all "active" jobs, but they are not well-rounded days of activity, nor do they help someone stay fit. In other words, keep in mind that even an active job doesn't make you "fit."

For example, if you are a nurse and are in stressful situations very often where you physically have to help people in and out of bed, you need to practice relaxation techniques and back, arm, chest, and core strengthening moves. You might also need to do aerobics to lose weight because even though you are on your feet, you're not actually moving enough to burn body fat. (You probably make 10,000 steps a day, but chances are you rarely get your heart rate up.)

Likewise, if you are a construction worker, you may already have strong arms and legs, but have you made sure that your back is strong so that when you lift heavy objects, your spine doesn't get sprained?

Although many people think personal trainers are a luxury, even a few sessions with a well-qualified one (see page 177) can give you a program tailored specifically to your needs. You should also check in with the trainer every few months to change your program enough to keep it interesting and in pace with your new fitness level.

Moving More

Think about when you sit without taking a break—in meetings, in front of the computer, when you're going through paperwork. All of these are times when you could move or stand instead of sitting. And, while everyone always suggests taking breaks, and while it often seems impossible if your job is busy or takes place in a company where taking breaks is frowned upon, know this: your health is suffering if you don't take breaks.

How to Take a Break

When you do get a break, be sure to make it an active one. Do not sit down at a table. Instead, walk. And preferably walk outside to get some fresh air. Walk fast. Even 10 minutes is enough for an interval session. Start to stroll and then, pick up the pace a little. You won't sweat and ruin your outfit, but you will feel much better and improve your metabolism and health.

If you've accepted your need for breaks, then there is one more step you can take, and that is to make your breaks truly active. While it's helpful to go outside and walk a bit, there are other things you can do to make your breaks even more effective. If you can't take a walk, use your 10-minute break to stretch.

If you do have a ball at your desk, use it for exercise. Roll over it (with your back on the ball) and let your chest stretch. Stand up and put your hands on the ball, then roll it out. Bring an exercise band to work and use it to stretch. You can do this sitting in your chair or standing up (much better, of course).

Joining a Gym

If you get a lunch hour, consider joining a gym near your office. Even if you have to walk or drive there, chances are you'll have at least 30 minutes to exercise, and with a gym, you'll have many workout options. Many gyms offer 30-minute lunch hour classes.

One issue with these classes is time for showering. If you work out hard enough, you'll sweat (or at least glow), and there's no getting around that. You can strive to create a routine where showering and getting redressed is possible. Lots of people do it (if you head to a gym at noon, you'll see that). But if you don't want to do that (and that's fine, don't berate yourself for that), accept that your workouts aren't going to be as intense as you need them to be, but do them anyway. Having an active lunch hour, even if it's moderate activity, is better than having a sedentary lunch hour.

Encouraging an Active Office

It's lunchtime and your coworkers (many of whom are most likely your friends, too), head over to a table to sit down, eat, and chat. Who wants to miss that? Certainly not you.

Peer pressure is a reality, especially when you want to hang with your buds. Here are some ways to recruit your coworkers to be more active:

- **Ask for support honestly.** Tell them you have a goal (you might even want to say it's on doctor's orders) to be more active during the day, and you'd like them to help you. Ask if they'd be interested in taking walks with you or in joining the gym.

- **Split up the fun.** Eat lunch with your friends on some days, and head to the gym on others. Don't think of the situation as win-lose; think of it as win-win—a compromise for you to do everything you enjoy.

If you sense resentment from your coworkers who haven't yet embraced the fit life, look for support elsewhere. Ask a friend or relative who does support your goals to call or e-mail you during the day to see how you are doing (just once; you don't have to waste a lot of time) so you don't feel alone.

It will only help your company, its employees, and your company's productivity if fitness—and therefore good health—is encouraged and supported. Call your health insurance provider and ask if they have any incentives for companies that promote health and wellness on their worksite. Then head to your human resources department and let them know about those incentives, since they might save the company money.

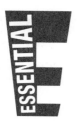

Health and fitness benefits are one of the measurements used to judge whether a company is good. Check out *Fortune, Money, Working Mother,* and other magazines that create those listings for "Best Places To Work"; all the top companies have onsite fitness. And while big changes may seem unlikely for a small company, small changes—such as buying exercise balls or providing everyone with exercise bands—will send an important and inexpensive message to employees: fitness is good for everyone.

Second, think about places in your company where something active, such as a Ping-Pong table, could be placed. Sound funny? Ping-Pong is physical and, believe it or not, it's one of the most common ways for a company to introduce some activity into their employees' lives.

Third, find the person in charge who likes to work out. Is it a VP who comes to the office straight from the gym every day? Does your CEO have a treadmill in his office? Go straight to that person (don't be afraid!) and explain that you want to help promote fitness in the workplace because it will reduce health insurance claims (and it will!) and make the office a more pleasant place to work.

If You Work at Home

With the proliferation of home computers and laptops, plenty of people are working at home, which means they sit more, and not just in chairs. You can work from your couch or recliner these days, too. Sitting in a chair at home for long periods of time—even if you're working—is just as detrimental to your posture and fitness as sitting in an office.

If you do work at home, follow the same advice as those in outside offices should take. Make your desk slightly inconvenient, don't sit for too long without getting up, and be sure you take some breaks. Also, be sure you're practicing good posture as you sit.

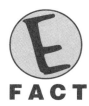

FACT

Home workers move even less than those who drive or walk to their offices. It's just common sense—they don't even have to get into or out of their car to start doing their work. If you work at home to cut your commute time, try to use some of that saved time to be active. And if you can, make it high-intensity activity so that it will contribute to your fitness level.

If you work at home, you'll also need to remember that there are times you can stand and move when other workers can't. For example, you can get a headset phone and walk when you're on a conference call. You can also stand at a desk or dresser to work, or work during a commute rather than sit. You can sit on an exercise ball rather than on a chair when you work, too.

Think Fitness, Not Comfort

Home workers are fortunate in that they can design their offices however they like, and it is possible to do this with fitness in mind. You can keep a treadmill in your office, or a set of free weights. Also, you can use an alarm clock to take 10-minute breaks, and make those breaks count by increasing their intensity as you get fitter. Remember, 10-minute bursts of activity are as effective as longer workouts at building health and, if you make those short workouts high intensity, they can also increase fitness.

Even if you don't have a treadmill or weights, use your breaks to run around your house, practice yoga, or do full-body resistance moves (shown in Chapter 7) to stay in shape.

Eating at Home

When you work at home, it's easy to snack on whatever's around, too, especially if you feel bored or lonely. Try to decide what you're going to eat before the day begins so that you won't be tempted by whatever's in the refrigerator when you're at home. And it's better if you can keep your favorite snack foods out of the house, since it's easy to hear those cookies and chips calling to when you're alone.

Fitness on the Road

A lot of business travelers complain that they can't get their regular exercise routine in when they are traveling for work. Most hotels have inferior gyms, with old treadmills and very little weight equipment. If you're going to travel for work, to stay in shape bring along a resistance band or some yoga or Pilates DVDs (you can run them on your laptop).

And remember, Tom Brokaw is famous for running up and down hotel stairs when he travel. You don't need machines to run or do other forms of exercise. Go outside, walk around, and see the sights where you're visiting. Practice good eating habits even when you travel; stay away from processed foods, and try to stop at grocery stores for fresh produce to make sure you're getting your nutrients from fruits and vegetables. You'll feel better when you travel, and look even better when you return home.

Chapter 15
Fitness Vacations

Traveling to a new destination coupled with being active is an exciting combination. How about running a 10k event in Hawaii or Florida? What about bicycling across your favorite state or European country? You could walk inn to inn in Spain or France. Or you can simply be sure the hotel you're staying in has a walking trail and a fitness room. And if you must go somewhere with no better options, then you'll know to at least head to your destination with the active intention to do jumping jacks and other cardio moves, as well as some resistance training with your own body weight.

Make Fitness Your Destination

As people are enjoying the travel-plus-physical-activity combination, there are more and more organized events and companies offering planned itineraries and official support. These organized events offer you the opportunity to go and see places you have never seen before, to be active in the great outdoors, and to meet new people while having fun.

Here are just a few destination events:

- Bay to Breakers, San Francisco, California
- Peachtree Road Race, Atlanta, Georgia
- Gasparilla Distance Classic, Tampa, Florida
- Bike Ride Around Lake Tahoe, Lake Tahoe, California
- Run to the Far Side, San Francisco, California

But that's thinking big. Your other option is to take an active vacation, with no goal other than to enjoy yourself, have fun, and not sit around. There is a dizzying array of trip options. They include spas with a fitness focus, resorts with activities (skiing, swimming, and skating), walking vacations, biking trips, hiking treks, and far more adventurous options, such as mountain climbing, backwoods cross-country snowshoeing, kayaking, trips during which you learn to sail, and other skill-focused trips. Whatever your trip, be sure to bring any equipment requested and the right shoes so that you'll be comfortable and able to take part in all of the activities available to you.

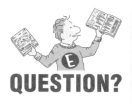

QUESTION?

Is relaxing forbidden on a fitness vacation?
No way! It can't be called a vacation if you don't spend some time resting and relaxing. You can choose, for example, to stay at a spa or resort that offers both pampering and activities. Or you can go all out and plan a trip around your favorite activity, such as walking or bicycling.

What if you're going to Disney World with your kids? Don't worry! You'll do a ton of walking at Disney World—and at most other amusement parks.

Getting from the hotel to the park and then going around the park practically guarantees that you'll walk more than you usually do throughout the day.

Also, if you're spending any amount of time at Disney World, you'll be staying at a nearby hotel, and those hotels usually have fitness rooms, although their usefulness is often sketchy (old machines and very few to choose from). But Disney World, like most other resorts, offers plenty of other activities for its visitors, such as horseback riding, swimming, and tennis.

If you want to strength train while you're traveling, consider packing a resistance band, or do a yoga routine or Pilates workout, or the strength-training routine in Appendix B.

The important thing to remember is that unlike the stereotype, most people do, in fact, lose weight on vacation. For one thing, they aren't sitting at a desk all day, so they are more active than usual. Second, just being more relaxed and having more fun—going out dancing at night or walking through museums—tends to lower stress hormones (which contribute to weight gain), and you burn more calories doing anything more than sitting in front of the TV at night.

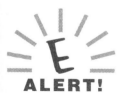

ALERT!

The biggest problem people have on vacation isn't their activity level, but the foods they eat. There is absolutely nothing wrong with having dessert, eating a little more of a special food, or even indulging in a junk food day when you're traveling. The point of a vacation is to have fun and relax. However, there are almost always ways to make sure you eat balanced, nutritious meals—plus treats—even while you're traveling.

Now, if you're traveling somewhere very remote or exotic, it is hard to eat anything other than what's common to the area in which you're staying. If you are going to faraway place, consider bringing jars of peanut butter as well as protein bars and dried fruit. These are nutritious and calorie-dense (so you won't get hungry), and won't spoil.

If you're on the road, think small portions, fresh food (grocery stores are everywhere) and balance (low-fat protein/veggies/whole grains and fruit, too). Drink plenty of water, too, of course.

Remember that even one or two weeks of unhealthy eating won't destroy your health or your fitness gains. Fun and a lack of stress and fretting are as important to your health as your diet.

Rather than worrying about gaining weight or losing your fitness level while you're on a trip, instead focus on ways to have fun and move more than you usually do. When planning your trip, make time for fitness, and you'll find that your trip is more fun.

Walking Trips

If you're considering a walking vacation, you need to ask yourself a couple of questions. First, how much walking do you do now, and second, how much do you want to do, and at what intensity, on a vacation?

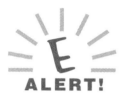

ALERT!

If you want to go on a walking vacation, find and wear comfortable, supportive walking shoes that you can train in, as well as vacation in. There is no bigger mistake that you can make than bringing new shoes on a walking vacation. You might even want to have two pairs: one with a rugged tread for trails, and one for walking on pavement.

Maybe you are someone who walks two miles every day. Here's a walking schedule to get ready for a walking vacation of four to five consecutive days of moderately paced, comfortable walking while sightseeing and enjoying the new surroundings. On average you'll walk 7 miles per day:

Week 1: Choose one interval, one endurance, one strength, and one freebie workout.

Weeks 2 and 3: Choose two interval, two endurance, one strength, and one freebie workout, but take one day off.

Week 4: Choose two interval, three endurance, and one strength workout, but take one day off.

Week 5: Choose one interval, four endurance, and two freebie workouts.

Week 6: Choose two endurance, one strength, two freebie workouts, but take two days off.

For this vacation, beginners especially, begin your training no less than six weeks prior.

Biking Vacations

Like walking trips, biking trips can range from the flat-terrained, gentle journeys from elegant inn to elegant inn, to the more strenuous hilly tours carrying a tent on your bicycle.

One good thing about bicycle trips is that you can cover a lot of ground (or at least more than you do when you walk) on your trip and, usually, you decide how much you ride each day. Most trip organizers have a van to carry luggage, food, and other necessities, so you can ride unencumbered and, if you get tired, they'll give you a lift in that van.

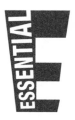

The organizers of biking trips will help you determine what level trip you should join. Serious cyclists will want to cover longer distances and will look for hills to climb, while the more leisurely cyclist should choose trips that are on flat ground or that offer some walking (the van will carry your bike) as well as riding.

If you are going to take a bicycle trip, be sure to get some rides in before you leave. Be aware of the distances you might be traveling on your trip, and try to get used to them. Also, see what accoutrements you need to be comfortable. While most bicycle-travel companies will provide you with a bike if you don't want to bring your own, do you want to bring a padded seat cover? Your own water bottles? A rearview mirror? Try to make your trip both comfortable and fun, which might mean dividing some of the preparation between you and the company hosting you.

Swimming on Vacation

These days, almost every hotel has a pool, which is great if you love to swim, but at the same time, terrible if you love to swim, because often the pools aren't maintained very well and are full of kids jumping around. And usually, the pools aren't shaped like your local lap pool.

If you are a swimmer and you want to swim on vacation, keep those warnings in mind as you book your hotel and pick your location. Some hotels have connections with nearby gyms so that you can find a more appropriate place for your workouts. Or you could call a local YMCA and see if they would give you a guest pass for the day.

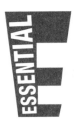

If you do end up being stuck at a hotel that has a pool shaped like a kidney, early-morning workouts will be your best bet. Kids rarely head to a pool before breakfast (because their parents don't), so you'll find it cleaner, quieter, and more conducive to working out effectively.

One great way to swim on vacation is, of course, to head to the nearest natural body of water. Don't assume, however, that lap swimming will translate exactly to your outdoor location. First, and foremost, remember that anyone who swims outside should never be alone. If you get tired or something happens, someone else needs to be within earshot.

Second, give yourself time to get used to your surroundings. During your first time in the ocean, lake, river, or bay, you shouldn't simply be focused on having fun. Is there a current? Do you need to consider the tides? Is what you have to swim with sufficient, or do you need a wetsuit or a bathing cap?

Third and finally, don't expect to swim for the same time and the same way as you do indoors. So, if you typically swim for an hour, don't be surprised if you're tired after 30 minutes. If you typically swim quickly, don't worry if you need to slow down. Different conditions present different challenges; rather than fight them, embrace them.

Keeping Your Cool

Looking forward to your vacation, but concerned that you'll lose any progress you've made and—horrors—gain weight? Don't worry. Here's what you need to do.

Be realistic. You're about to take a vacation, and a vacation from your workout schedule is as beneficial as a vacation from work and household chores. So, give yourself permission to enjoy yourself and lounge for a little while. Even with a few days off, you won't lose any strength or cardio gains you've made. However, after a few weeks, the story changes.

Figure out how you are going to get some exercise at some point, especially if you're on a long vacation. Don't try to mimic your workout exactly; it's rare to be somewhere with the same equipment or walking paths. Instead, be creative and open to options. If you typically walk, you might need to ride the stationary cycle in the fitness room. If you usually use free weights, you might be able to figure out how to use the weight-training station in the fitness room.

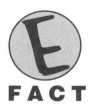

FACT

On vacation, you won't be an active person (well, not most likely), but you can enjoy and watch sports, which is very inspirational. You might want to attend the Olympic Games or Olympic Trials, the Boston Marathon, Ironman Triathlons, the Special Olympics, or the Tour de France.

Think about your diet. Do not, under any circumstances, refuse to enjoy a treat or have a snack. Eating well is not about deprivation; it is about balance and moderation. So recognize that you're going to enjoy some special desserts or an afternoon of chips in front of the TV, and enjoy it while it's happening. Then go back to your regular, healthy, fitness-oriented life.

Adventure Vacations

For bold travelers, there's nothing more exciting than an adventure vacation. Not only do you get to experience a place you've never seen before, but also you get to challenge yourself physically and keep in shape. This type of vacation can go in many directions. Are you interested in biking? Perhaps you'd like to bike through France, stopping at hostels along the way. Do you like running in races? Why not follow a trail of 5K races all over New England in the spring?

Here are some other ideas that might fulfill your adventurous whims. Web sites for these trips are listed in Appendix A:

- Walk the outback of Australia
- Learn to surf in Hawaii
- Learn to sail in the British Virgin Islands
- Bicycle through Baja California
- Hike to Machu Picchu
- Helihike in British Columbia

The important thing to remember about these trips is that they require training. Even if you're very active, you need to train specifically, i.e., train for the type of trip you're going to take. Ask the group you're going with to advise you on ways you can get in shape to get the most out of your trip.

Make Any Vacation Active

While adventurous vacations are lots of fun and give you great memories, they can take a lot of planning and money. If you don't have the means or the stamina for such a vacation, don't worry! You can turn almost any vacation into a fitness vacation with just a few easy additions. The following is a list of things you should consider taking with you on your trip, although, of course, the exact list will depend on your location and activity:

- Sneakers
- Exercise bands
- An iPod with downloaded workout programs
- Workout clothes
- Exercise DVDs
- Bathing suit, towel, bathing cap, goggles
- Yoga mat
- Bike shorts

And finally, last but not least, if you want to consider luxury with fitness, consider fitness spas! Spas used to be associated with weight loss and deprivation, but now they have not only accepted but embraced the knowledge that fitness is an essential part of health, weight loss, and relaxation. Spas will encourage you now to hike, swim, lift weights, and do Pilates and yoga, and you can do any of these things in Arizona, Tennessee, or Provence! See Appendix A for a list of fitness spas.

Chapter 16

Sleep and Stress

People often like to brag that not only do they not get any sleep, they don't need any sleep. They may get more work done at the office or read more books, but chances are that they're not in good health. Look closely at these people. Are they energetic? Perky? Healthy looking? Probably not. No matter how lame it may seem to go to bed early and get a good night's sleep, it's incredibly important to your health. Sleep translates into health, happiness, and even weight loss.

The Need for Sleep

Sleep is something we need, and without it, our bodies and our minds do not function properly. There is no substitute for sleep, and to deny its necessity, to deny how much you need it, is to not take care of yourself.

Your body, including your brain, actually mends and maintains itself when you sleep. If you strength train or do any sort of resistance exercise, then your muscles repair themselves and grow stronger when you're asleep. If you don't sleep, your muscles will stay fatigued and not get stronger. Getting enough sleep helps keep you safe; being sleep-deprived increases the likelihood of accidents and mistakes. If you want to stay healthy—have fewer colds, for example—keep in mind that not getting enough sleep will lower your immune system so you'll be more likely to get sick, and stay sick longer.

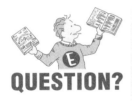

QUESTION?

How do I know if I'm not sleeping enough?
If you fall asleep as you're watching TV or when you are a passenger in a car, there is a good chance you don't sleep enough. Other signs of sleep deprivation include feeling your energy drop significantly in the late afternoon, not being able to stay awake when lights go out for a meeting or the movies, or not being able to stay focused during conversations, as if you're drifting off.

It's all about moderation when it comes to sleep. If you have been sleeping more than nine or ten hours or have trouble getting out of bed in the morning even after a full night's sleep, then you may be suffering from depression or another illness, with fatigue as a symptom. Sleeping too much is definitely something about which you should speak to your doctor, because, it, too, will prevent you from getting fit and losing weight.

Sleeping Your Way Toward Weight Loss

If you're trying to lose weight, sleep helps your body regulate itself so that your hormones and metabolism function properly. If you don't sleep enough, you might crave food and eat for energy (to stay awake). But more than that, your body won't help you lose weight if you're tired. Your metabolism will slow down, your hormones will go kerflooey, and weight loss? It won't be as likely to happen, or it won't happen as quickly as it could.

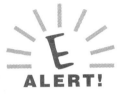

ALERT!

You might sacrifice sleep to get more done during the day, believing that you are so busy you can't afford to take eight or nine hours out of your schedule, but a restful night has been shown to make you more productive and energetic during the day. In other words, sleep is actually beneficial to a busy person.

Of course, millions of us don't sleep enough or, if we do sleep enough hours, we don't get enough quality sleep. We toss and turn, or wake up too often during the night.

It's not okay to just pop a sleeping pill, because that isn't actually fixing the problem; it's ignoring a symptom. In other words, if you're not sleeping well, then something else is going on, and when you fix that, you'll sleep better.

The Reasons Behind Insufficient Sleep

Chances are, you know why you can't sleep. When the lights go out, you worry about your relationship or your job, your neighbor plays his stereo all night, or your kid sleeps with you and kicks you. But if you are having trouble figuring out what's keeping you awake, here are some possibilities to consider.

Environmental Irritations

Noise, light, an uncomfortable bed. If you're not comfortable, you're not going to sleep well, and what makes you comfortable is personal. You might prefer to sleep in a room that's pitch black or has a nightlight, or you might enjoy soothing music or a book before bed. If you're not sure what will put you to sleep and keep you asleep, then you need to experiment and see what works. Then stick with it.

Eating Before Bed

You might be eating too much before bed. Or you could be eating too little. Too much food keeps you awake because your body has to work to digest it, which makes you physically busy, i.e., unable to rest. Too little food, on the other hand, makes you hungry, and your body wants to eat before it wants to sleep, i.e., food takes precedence over sleep, so hunger can keep your eyes open.

Lots of people restrict their food intake too much during the day and then eat semi-uncontrollably at night. It's because they're hungry. If you wake up at a reasonable hour and eat breakfast—a real breakfast, not just coffee and a doughnut—then you'll actually improve your sleep.

Caffeine and Alcohol

Soda, iced tea, sports drinks (Red Bull, for example, contains caffeine), and alcohol can disrupt your sleep, even though alcoholic drinks may help you fall asleep initially. If you're going to have a cocktail before bed, make sure it's at least three or four hours before your head hits the pillow. And if you are in the habit of enjoying an afternoon cup of coffee, make it decaf or, even better, try to cut it out altogether.

Medicine or Drugs

Any chemical that you ingest, even pot or an over-the-counter painkiller, can alter your sleep pattern. Sometimes that can work for you (if you have a headache, then an over-the-counter pain remedy can let you sleep), but other times medicine or drugs can make you jittery. Some painkillers even have very high levels of caffeine in them, so read the label.

Tension

Worried? Nervous? Lonely? Sad? Sometimes we keep ourselves awake by thinking too much. Letting go of your thoughts so that your mind can rest is necessary for sleep. But in fact, many of us are never taught how to go to sleep as children, and so we struggle as adults to find ways to relax. If something is bothering you, get out a journal and a pen, and write down your concerns. If you are still worried and your thinking keeps you up for several nights in a row, consider talking to someone to work through and resolve the issue.

Hormones

Hormones—can't live without 'em, can't go to sleep when they're raging. Women typically find that their sleep pattern changes throughout their monthly cycle, and change even more when they are premenopausal, menopausal, and postmenopausal. Recognizing the cause of your lack of sleep—which you can usually do simply by ruling out the typical problems listed above—can also point you in the direction of possible solutions.

Help Yourself Sleep Better

Each of the problems listed so far in this chapter has a potential solution, of course, but before we get into specifics, it's helpful to first recognize that you want to sleep well, i.e, seven to nine hours of interrupted sleep each night. Just setting that intention (you read about intention setting in Chapter 1) will help you get on the path to a good night's sleep.

Go to sleep and wake up at the same times. Your body loves regularity. If you are someone who sleeps very late on the weekends and then has trouble waking up for work on Monday, or if you sometimes stay up late and then crash the next evening, you aren't helping yourself. Instead, figure out what time you need to wake up on most days. Let's say it's 6:30. Count back eight hours (seven if you're used to going to bed late) and plan to be in bed at 10:30. Do whatever it is you need to do so that you're in bed at that time (brush your teeth, wash up, be in pajamas, etc.). Then once you're in bed, put on some music if you want, turn off the lights, and close your eyes. If after 15 minutes you are still awake, read for a little bit. Just try to stay in bed and relax.

At 10:30 P.M. the next night, start the whole process again. Within a few nights you should be sleeping well. If you're not, go through the list above and try to figure out what the problem is. Are you drinking too much coffee? Worried about the next day's appointments? Work on each possible issue as you need to, but stick to the sleeping schedule, give or take a half hour or so, based on your sleep needs (maybe you do only need seven hours, or maybe you need nine). Getting regular, good sleep may take a few weeks of planning and adjustment, but the rewards are amazing in terms of energy, mood, and health.

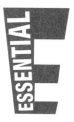

No matter what time you actually fall asleep, get out of bed and into sunlight (even if you just stand in front of a window) at 6:30. Try to exercise a little, too, at 6:30. Do some stretches, some yoga, or even dance to the radio. The combination of light and activity will start to set your internal clock, which will encourage better sleep.

Napping

Napping during the day is great for some people, but only if your nap lasts for less than a half hour (10 to 15 minutes is perfect for most people). If your naps last too long, then they may interfere with your nighttime sleep, but at the same time, they might not be long enough to truly be restful. This is especially true if you're taking naps when you should be doing something else, such as working.

What to Do When You Aren't Sleeping

Of course, even the best sleepers sometimes have sleepless nights. If you are someone who typically sleeps well but occasionally finds yourself awake at 3:00 A.M., try not to stress about it. Get out of bed and clean the kitchen. Do a load of laundry. Try to be easily active without turning on a lot of lights or doing something that requires a lot of thought. You can even take a shower. The heat may help you feel tired.

You also can consider having a snack. In fact, you might try having this snack a few hours before bed if your insomnia continues. The snack, however, has to be specific. It should include a little bit of low-fat protein (e.g., a slice of cheese or a tablespoon of cottage cheese) and more complex carbs, such as a serving of whole-grain cracker or a slice of whole-wheat bread.

Other foods that help you sleep are those rich in the B vitamins, such as peas and lima beans. Also, people who don't eat enough iron, calcium, and other minerals are thought to have sleep problems, so if you're having trouble sleeping, strive for a balanced diet throughout the day, and see if that helps.

Also consider that you might not be able to sleep because something is on your mind. If this is the case, get out of bed, put a low light on, get out some paper and a pen, and start writing. Write out everything that comes in your head—what's worrying you and what you think you might want to do about it. Keep writing until you have nothing left to say.

If the same thing happens the following night, then promise yourself you will share your worries with someone. Often, just getting your feelings out will help you feel better, but if your sleeplessness lasts over a couple of days, it may be time to talk about what's on your mind.

Try not to let your worries get in the way of your health and wellness, because you can take charge of your concerns. Expressing yourself and finding someone who will listen and support you can give you back your rest. The good news about talking out your problems is that not only will you sleep better, but you might also find a way to fix what's worrying you in the first place.

Stress

These days stress doesn't come typically come from life-threatening situations; instead you feel stressed when your baby is crying but you have work to do and your phone is ringing. You want to exercise, but you have a project due, and your husband wants to go out. Stress occurs when you have too much to do, and too little time to do it. Or when you have a problem and you can't figure out a solution or feel powerless to fix it. These days, a lot of stress takes place in our head—worry—rather than in a physical situation, such as danger.

Your body best handles short-term stress, but society delivers the long-term type, where adrenaline forces more blood through your vessels without giving your heart the strength to deal with it. This, in turn, raises your risk of stroke and heart disease. In response, your body releases the hormone cortisol, which stores fatty acids in the form of adipose tissue around your belly.

Stress is a cycle of mental and then physical problems, which, in turn, lead to another concern or worry. Learning how to effectively manage stress will help you sleep better, remain fitter and healthier, and give you more tools to handle the inevitable struggles inherent in work and relationships.

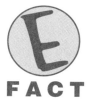

FACT

Your worries are real, but your response to those concerns can make things worse. You need to find effective ways to manage your life so that your stress doesn't get out of hand and begin to take over the rest of your life, such as time with your family, sleep time, your job, or workout time.

You don't feel stress when you're at the office or taking care of your child because your mind is absorbed by a task. Instead, we worry about things when we should be sleeping and when, in the middle of the night, we really can't do much about whatever the problem is, be it bills or relationship fears. Or the stress stops you from being present at work or with your child because it's so overwhelming that you can't stop thinking about it.

Stress Reducers

Exercise is, of course, a great stress reducer. When your body functions at a high level, your brain is more likely to be able to think of creative solutions to your problems as well as be able to stay calm even if you're concerned about something. The important thing to remember is that stress and stressful feelings, such as worry, obsessive thinking, or crying, also don't solve problems. Your problem is real, and reducing stress doesn't mean ignoring what's on your mind—but it does mean learning to keep your mind and body calm when you have a concern.

Slow Down Your Breath

When stress gets a hold of your mind and your body, you probably start to take shallower breaths. So, if you can, consciously try to slow down your breathing, focusing on lengthening your inhales and exhales and bringing the oxygen down deep into your body. This breathing technique will reduce your heart rate as well as soothe the natural stress response of your body.

Take a Walk or Do Something Repetitive

Very often when we're stressed, we think obsessively about what's worrying us, such as bills or a relationship. However, as mentioned previously, this obsessive thought is not only disturbing, it's not useful, and rarely helps us find a solution to our problem.

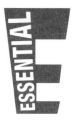

Crosswords, word-search puzzles, Sudoku, and other puzzles are all good ways to occupy your mind without stressing it. These activities will keep your brain fit, too. Just try to find puzzles that match your skill level. Puzzles that are too difficult will add stress, not reduce it!

Instead of worrying endlessly, take a walk, enjoy a shower, or do something repetitive, such as knitting or crocheting. Keeping part of your brain occupied with a repetitive action actually frees up the creative side of your brain to solve problems. This is why we often have great ideas when we are in the shower or not thinking about something in particular.

Do a Mind-body Routine

Yoga, Pilates, stretching, and other mind-body exercises relax the mind as well as the body by helping link movement to the breath, which, in turn, stops the physical response to stress. If you find yourself worried about something, try doing some yoga (revisit Chapter 10 for a refresher) or taking a few minutes to stretch, even if it's in the middle of the night. This gentle level of activity can burn off the physical tension, relax your muscles, and, at the same time, keep your worrying brain from obsessing about a concern for too long.

Laugh

Although TV can keep you up when you should be sleeping, laughing at a TV show or movie can do a lot to physically and mentally refocus your mind away from stress. If you do watch TV at night when you can't sleep, try something funny or mindless, as opposed to a documentary or a serious movie.

Remember, stress reduction doesn't mean that your worries aren't real, or that you are ignoring your problems. It only means that you are finding useful solutions to your problems while reducing the impact stress has on your body and spirit.

Chapter 17
Eating Right

Few of us past the age of five or so eat for the right reasons, which is to say for energy and health. When we are six, for example, we might eat because we are told to or because the candy dish is in front of us. Then, as we get older, we try not to eat because we think not eating is the way to stay thin. Eventually, if we are lucky, we begin to eat foods that are nutritious as well as foods that we like just for the fun in it, in the proper amounts.

Eating for Fitness

It takes a while for most of us to learn to eat properly. Let's face it: between emotional eating; the unhealthy products that pass for food that so many of us find in our cafeterias, offices, and grocery stores; the time we don't have (or think we don't have) for cooking; plus the neurotic messages we get about weight from the media and our families, it is difficult to learn to eat well, much less to actually eat well. Most of us eat to feel good, or we eat because the food around us is convenient, or we eat because it's time to eat, i.e., we've been told to eat three meals a day, plus snacks, and so that's what we try to do.

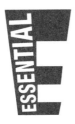

When you eat properly, you will keep your weight in check, build muscle, and maintain your metabolism. Your mood will be regulated, and you will think clearly. Your energy level will be up and steady. Your skin will be clear, your eyes bright, and your hair healthy. Eating properly also fights osteoporosis, type 2 diabetes, and brain degeneration. It can moderate PMS and other hormonal issues, promote good sleep, and support your immune system so you are less likely to get sick.

When you're eating for fitness, though, you have specific aims. First, you want to make sure what you eat gives you steady energy and won't interfere with your workouts. Second, you want to make sure the calories you eat are nutrient dense, i.e., that the foods you eat have plenty of vitamins and minerals.

A *calorie* is a unit of energy. Every calorie you eat translates into a calorie you can use, or burn (we often say "burn calories" because calories are kind of like a fire in that they provide your body with heat or energy). You burn, for example, about 40 calories an hour watching TV. Empty-calorie foods are those that often have a high number of calories, but those calories aren't nutritious, so they can pack on pounds and give you energy but don't help your body become and remain healthy.

Now, consider that many people eat ice cream when they watch TV. A bowl of ice cream is about 400 calories. You are taking in 400 calories and burning 40 calories an hour.

You see the immediate problem: you're taking in more calories than you're burning.

The second problem, though, is that most ice-cream calories aren't nutritious. Yes, there's calcium, but other than that, there is a high amount of fat and very little fiber, vitamins, minerals, or antioxidants. If you were striving to eat a nutrient-dense diet and still wanted to eat 400 calories, you could have, for instance, tomato (40 calories) and carrots (30 calories), sprouts (25 calories), grilled chicken (200 calories), and a glass of red wine (90 calories). And if you wanted to splurge and still get a hit of something rich and decadent (like the ice cream), you could have 2 ounces of dark chocolate.

Now, you'll notice that the second meal is, just that, a meal, while the ice cream is a snack. Also, even if you know almost nothing about nutrition, you know that the vegetables and chicken are better for you than the ice cream. Finally, you might notice that the second meal is larger and probably more satisfying than the ice cream by itself.

Foods You Need

Nutrition—the science of food and its effect on our bodies—is pretty new, at least in comparison to other sciences. But at this point, the science has singled out about forty specific nutrients, each of which has a purpose. Each nutrient is a chemical that fulfills one of three functions in the body: gives you energy, helps grow and repair tissue, or regulates your metabolism.

Nutrients include water, vitamins, and minerals, which grow and repair tissue; and carbohydrates, fat, and protein, which give you energy by providing calories. All of the nutrients regulate your metabolism by helping your body function smoothly and in balance.

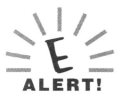

The most important thing to remember is that every nutrient is important, and the idea that you need to cut out fat, or carbs, or any other nutrient for that matter, is just wrong. The best eating plans balance nutrients and utilize the healthiest ones, but all nutrients are important and have a job to do, so cutting any one of them out completely is not good for your health or your fitness.

Food News

As everyone knows, the news is filled with reports about food that is good for you and a food that is bad for you, and those two foods are often the same. As nutritional research develops, so does the advice we get. For example, an egg has protein (in the white part) and fat (in the yellow part), but no carbohydrates. The white has few other nutrients, while the yellow has a high amount of vitamin B12 and folate. Nutritionists used to think that because the yellow part held all the fat, it wasn't good to eat too many yolks, but now they know that the fat in an egg is good for the brain and doesn't contribute to higher levels of cholesterol in the blood.

Likewise, even though this section of the book covers nutrients, the fact is, we think about eating food, not specific chemicals. So, it's much more helpful to think about eating nutritious foods than to think about giving ourselves specific nutrients.

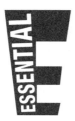

It's quite possible that we know only the tip of the iceberg when it comes to nutrition. For example, ten years ago no one knew that dark chocolate contains antioxidants, which are good for you. Instead, everyone assumed that because chocolate contains a high amount of saturated fat, it wasn't nutritious.

So it's best to keep this general rule in mind: eat moderate amounts, and eat a wide variety of whole foods rather than processed foods. Just following that one rule will be enough to help you make wiser meal choices.

Calorie Types and Body Weight

Your body does not discriminate based upon the types or source of calories. For example, when you eat, it doesn't matter whether the calories consumed are high fat, low fat, or nonfat. The bottom line is you have taken in more calories. When the body accumulates an excess of 3,500 calories (in other words, calories that are not being used), it will store them as one pound of fat regardless of whether they are from carbohydrates, fat, or protein. In terms of storage and weight gain or loss, a calorie is a calorie.

Where do calories come from? Calories come from only carbohydrates, fats, and proteins, not from vitamins or minerals. And each of these three nutrients (carbohydrates, fats, and proteins) has its own energy value.

Nutrients

As mentioned previously, proteins, carbohydrates, and fat all provide calories to the body. Foods also contain the nutrients that build and repair cells, including vitamins and minerals. Within each of those categories are subdivisions. For example, there are twenty-two amino acids in proteins; different types of fat, such as saturated and monounsaturated; and there are complex and simple carbohydrates.

Protein

Proteins, which are made up of amino acids, are considered the cell's building blocks for all tissues and cells in the body, including red blood cells, muscle, and hair. A secondary function of protein is to be an energy provider, a backup to carbohydrates. No matter what food it's found in, one gram of protein equals four calories. Protein is found in meat, fish, dairy products (cheeses, milk, yogurt), and legumes (beans and peas).

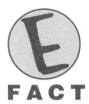

FACT

A study published in *The American Journal of Clinical Nutrition* found that when people ate more protein and cut down on fat they also reduced their calorie intake by 441 calories a day. In fact, experts think that eating protein enhances the effect of leptin, a hormone that helps the body feel full.

Legumes are excellent sources of protein; they are high in fiber and low in fat. Animal sources of protein are usually high in fat, although the type of fat and its amount varies widely (you'll read more about fat in a minute). Protein is essential to people who want to get strong and who want to lose weight.

Carbohydrates

One gram of carbohydrates always has four calories. Carbohydrates, sometimes called carbs, should make up 55 to 60 percent of the total calories consumed. The majority of these calories should come from complex carbohydrates. Sugars and starches are carbohydrates, and both of these fuel our brain and muscles. Their primary function is to supply energy quickly. Fiber is also a carbohydrate, but our bodies don't digest it.

Complex Carbohydrates

Complex carbohydrates are long connected chains of molecules that are chemically more complex than simple carbohydrates. Complex carbs are found in vegetables, beans, grains, and pasta. They take longer to enter the bloodstream because they are complex and thus take longer to break down into absorbable sugars. Complex carbohydrates are high in fiber, low in calories (compared to fat and alcohol), and low in fat; they have a longer life span than simple carbs, which keeps your energy level up for lengthy periods of time, and give a contented feeling of fullness. They are stored in the liver and muscles as glycogen.

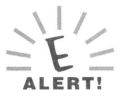

ALERT!

Don't count grams of nutrients. Instead, think about your meals. Here's the ideal proportion of your food intake: Get 55 to 60 percent of your calories from carbs, 30 percent from protein, and 20 percent from fat—the pounds will come off without you doing any other counting.

Simple Carbohydrates

Molecularly simple, with their single or double sugar molecules, means they release quickly into the bloodstream but have a short life span. They are found in some fruits, processed sugar, and processed foods. When simple carbs come in the form of processed foods, they are usually lower in fiber and higher in calories than complex carbohydrates.

Like all other calories, calories from carbs are stored as fat only if you eat too many of them, i.e. too many calories in general. And stay away from processed carbs. Studies have shown that the more processed food someone eats, the more they weigh.

Fats

Even though you hear a lot of bad things about fat, it is a necessary nutrient—in the right amounts! Fat supplies essential fatty acids, an important source of energy for aerobic exercise. Free fatty acids make up the main fuel for muscles at rest and during light activity. Stored fat in the body is important for protecting vital organs, insulating against cold, and transporting fat-soluble vitamins (A, D, E, and K). There are two types of fats, saturated and unsaturated.

Saturated Fats

Saturated fats are the "bad fats." These are found in animal foods and products (like beef, pork, ham, and sausage); dairy products, especially whole dairy products (like whole milk, cheese, cream, ice cream); and oils (like coconut oil, cottonseed oil, and palm kernel oils). They are typically solid at room temperature.

Trans Fatty Acids (TFAs), or Hydrogenated Vegetable Oils

Although not officially considered saturated fats, trans fatty acids are included with the saturated fats for a good reason. The body responds to TFAs as if they were saturated fats, the harmful kind that raises cholesterol and increases your risk of heart disease. When manufacturers recognized that they could improve the shelf life, flavor, and profit of their processed foods by hydrogenating (adding hydrogen to) polyunsaturated oils, such as corn or vegetable oil, they couldn't act fast enough. Hydrogenation turns polyunsaturated oils into solids.

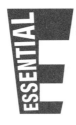

Nuts are high in fat but amazingly good for you. They have minerals, fiber, and nice amounts of protein. A great snack food, nuts should be eaten in moderation because they are high in calories; think of a serving as a tablespoon or two. Look for nuts that are unsalted; it's not important whether they are roasted or unroasted. Nuts are great sprinkled on foods high in vitamin C, such as fruit and vegetables, because the vitamin C increases the body's absorption of the iron in nuts.

Read your packaged food labels carefully; if you eat foods that have TFAs, include them in your saturated fat count. Unfortunately, they are not yet accounted for on the nutrition-facts panel along with the saturated fats, but will be in a few years. You have to look for them in the ingredients listing, where they are listed as partially hydrogenated vegetable (or other) oils. The most commonly used hydrogenated oil is soybean oil. TFAs are found in manufactured cookies, crackers, and fried foods.

Unsaturated Fats

Unsaturated fats are the preferred fats, although they should not be consumed above the recommended level. The two types of unsaturated fats are monounsaturated and polyunsaturated. Monounsaturated fats are found in olive and canola oils. They are touted as the healthiest of the oils. Polyunsaturated fats are found in corn, safflower, soybean, and sunflower oils.

Foods You Don't Need

There is a very easy way to know what foods you shouldn't eat: if it's not real, don't eat it. Pork rinds. Breakfast bars. Toaster pastries. Let's face it, Americans have their own—interesting—way of believing that certain manufactured (and yet tasty) products are actually food, i.e., what your body needs to give it energy as well as vitamins, minerals, and other nutrients so that your body keeps running smoothly and you keep being healthy.

But, guess what? Toaster pastries aren't food. Yes, some of the ingredients are food—or once were food before the nutrients were processed out of them—but, for the most part, the ingredients in toaster pastries and manufactured products like them aren't really food.

The thing is, nothing else tastes quite like a toaster pastry, and if you're someone who feels like she has to have her toaster pastries—and yet still wants to keep her weight at a manageable level—then you have to figure out how to make these items a once-in-a- while treat, or substitute a healthy food.

For example, let's say you typically eat a toaster pastry because it's quick and tastes sweet. Well, you could instead have whole-wheat toast, butter, and sliced strawberries. The nutritional difference is substantial, but the preparation time isn't really that different. To save even more time, in the time it takes to toast the bread, you can slice the strawberries.

In other words, eat real food, not "food" that was created in a factory and by a manufacturer. Plan to eat food rather than food products, and there is a good chance your weight and your health will benefit from it.

Now, this doesn't mean you can't eat fun foods, but it's better to eat foods that come from natural products, such as a real brownie, rather than a snack cake that comes in a box. If you can, cook and bake yourself so you know exactly what's going into your food. Read cookbooks and learn how to make healthy substitutions. For example, applesauce is a great substitute for butter when you bake.

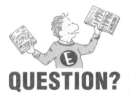

I can't stand to cut out all of my treats from my diet. What are some healthier but still-tasty alternatives?

To have a healthy lifestyle, you don't have to eliminate everything you enjoy. If you typically have a candy bar every afternoon at three, then instead you could have a small square of dark chocolate (again, there are high amounts of antioxidants in that), and some nuts and raisins with it. Or, if you're someone who can't resist treats like pastrami, pepperoni, or salami, i.e., salty meats, then you could have a healthy protein option instead, such as a lean piece of turkey or sliced chicken.

All-important Water

Water is perhaps the most important of the six essential nutrients. You may be able to survive for many days and even weeks without food, but not so with water. Drinking water because it is a vital nutrient is reason enough to consume it regularly. But water also has many specific jobs in the body, including transporting nutrients, gases, and waste products, regulating body heat, and soothing and moistening. Water is found in food and fluids. The human body is approximately 60 to 70 percent water. It is one of the major ingredients of your anatomy and is necessary for an optimum physiological environment.

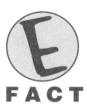

FACT

Signs that you may not be drinking enough water include bad breath, a pasty mouth or tongue, dark colored or smelly urine, intestinal cramping, diarrhea or constipation, dry skin, and headaches. But don't worry: water isn't the only fluid that can hydrate you. Other options include herbal teas, juice, soy or rice beverages, and milk.

How do you know if you are getting enough water? Daily, you want to drink a minimum of 64 ounces (more than five twelve-ounce glasses) of water, plus other hydrating fluids. Hydrating fluids are nonalcoholic, noncaffeinated, and don't have added sugar. If you drink 64 ounces of water daily and do not have any signs of dehydration, you probably are getting enough water. But when you notice the signs that you're drinking too little, add some water to your diet. Water is a very simple remedy to some pretty unpleasant conditions.

Even though they are made with water, alcoholic, caffeinated, and carbonated beverages dehydrate the body, or cause it to lose fluid. If you consume those beverages, compensate with a 1:1 ratio of water for each one of those you consume. If you consume those beverages habitually, you might consider replacing them with water and a variety of the other hydrating beverages.

One of the simplest actions you can take toward improving your nutrition is to drink plenty of fluids. Having a conscious plan will help you to drink the recommended amount. Start your day with a twelve- to twenty-ounce water wake-up call. If you are a coffee or tea drinker, have some water by itself first. The water sets you up to be hydrated from the beginning of the day, gently wakes up your body, and helps stimulate your bowels naturally.

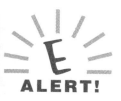

ALERT!

Alcohol is a depressant, so even though it makes you loose for a while, in the long run it brings you down. Alcohol slows your reaction time, packs a caloric punch (7 calories per gram; fat has 9 calories per gram), and dehydrates you.

Buy (or pick from your cupboard) a nice water bottle and prefill it with water so that you have a visual reminder that you need to drink. Plan to drink the water in it before lunchtime or before you leave the office. Keep a full bottle in your car, on your bike, or in your backpack, and drink it before you reach your destination. If you work in an office, keep refilling the bottle at the water cooler. Have a cutoff time when you stop drinking, typically a couple of hours prior to sleep, so your bladder will not be vying for your attention while you are trying to sleep.

Vitamins and Minerals

Vitamins are compounds that help the body perform many functions. Here are just some of the good reasons why you want to eat a variety of wholesome foods and take in a wide range of vitamins:

- Vitamin A is a moisturizer for your skin and mucous membranes. It also aids vision. Sources include carrots, sweet potatoes, margarine, butter, and liver.
- Vitamin B1 (thiamin) works with other enzymes to help you extract energy from carbohydrates. Sources include whole grains, nuts, and lean pork.
- Vitamin B2 (riboflavin) is a coenzyme and does work similar to vitamins A and B1. Sources include milk, yogurt, and cheese.
- Vitamin B3 (niacin) facilitates energy production in cells. Sources include lean meat, fish, poultry, and grains.
- Vitamin B6 (pyroxdine) absorbs and metabolizes protein and aids in red-blood-cell formation. Sources include lean meat, vegetables, and whole grains.
- Vitamin B12 (cobalamin) is involved in the synthesis of nucleic acids and red blood cell formation. Sources include meats, milk products, and eggs.
- Biotin is a coenzyme in the synthesis of fatty acids and glycogen formation. Sources include egg yolks and dark green vegetables.
- Folic acid (folacin) functions as a coenzyme in the synthesis of nucleic acids and protein. Sources include green vegetables, beans, and whole-wheat products.
- Vitamin C is responsible for intracellular maintenance of bone, the capillaries, and teeth. Sources include citrus fruits, green peppers, and tomatoes.
- Vitamin D aids in the formation and growth of bones and teeth; it also promotes calcium absorption. Sources include eggs, tuna, liver, and fortified milk.
- Vitamin E supports the immune system and prevents cell-membrane damage. Sources include vegetable oils, whole-grain cereal and bread, and leafy green vegetables.

- Vitamin K is important in blood clotting. Sources include leafy green vegetables, peas, and potatoes.

Minerals are inorganic substances that help the body perform many functions. Here are some highlights:

- Calcium gives support to bones, teeth, blood clotting, and nerve and muscle function. Sources include milk, sardines, dark green vegetables, and nuts.
- Chloride facilitates nerve and muscle function and water balance (with sodium). Sources include table salt.
- Chromium aids glucose metabolism. Sources include meats, liver, whole grains, and dried beans.
- Copper supports enzyme function and energy production. Sources include meats, seafood, nuts, and grains.
- Iodine facilitates thyroid hormone formation. Sources include iodized salt and seafood.
- Iron helps in oxygen transport in red blood cells and enzyme function. Sources include red meat, liver, eggs, beans, leafy vegetables, and shellfish.
- Magnesium aids bone growth and nerve, muscle, and enzyme function. Sources include nuts, seafood, whole grains, and leafy green vegetables.
- Manganese supports enzyme function. Sources include whole grains, nuts, fruits, and vegetables.
- Phosphorus helps bone, teeth, and energy transfer. Sources include meats, poultry, seafood, eggs, milk, and beans.
- Potassium facilitates nerve and muscle function. Sources include fresh vegetables, bananas, cantaloupe, citrus fruits, milk, meats, and fish.
- Selenium works with vitamin E. Sources include meat, fish, whole grains, and eggs.
- Sodium aids nerve and muscle function and water balance. Sources include table salt.
- Zinc aids in enzyme function and growth. Sources include meat, shellfish, yeast, and whole grains.

For women, one of the most important minerals is calcium. The disease osteoporosis, a softening of the bones, has spotlighted the need for adequate daily calcium intake. This important mineral helps keep your bones strong. The daily recommended intake for calcium is 1000 milligrams per day. Even if you plan to take a calcium supplement (calcium citrate is recommended), you will want to get at least half of your calcium from food sources. Finally, when eating dairy products, use the low-fat or nonfat varieties. Even though most of the fat has been removed from low-fat skim milk and yogurt (not frozen), they retain all the calcium and protein.

Dietary Fiber

Dietary fiber comes from substances found in the walls of plant cells that the body cannot digest. There are two types of fiber, insoluble and soluble. The recommendation for daily dietary fiber intake is 25 to 35 grams, and if you currently eat less, you should increase your fiber intake gradually. You will notice the difference when you have more fiber in your diet. The indigestibility of fiber, especially insoluble fiber, helps prevent you from overeating because it gives you a feeling of fullness. But even more importantly, fiber works wonders on your digestive tract.

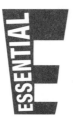

Fiber is lost during food processing, so when possible eat the less-processed version of a food. Juicing fruits, pureeing vegetables, and removing edible skins off fruits and vegetables are all manufacturing processes that reduce fiber. It is recommended that you eat a variety of fiber-rich foods so that you get enough of both types of fiber, insoluble and soluble.

Insoluble fiber traveling through the digestive tract acts like a magnet and sponge, attracting and absorbing water and digested food to form fecal matter. This water softens and adds weight to the stool, which helps facilitate its transit time. Insoluble fibers such as those found in wheat bran and other grains, fruits, and vegetables help to prevent hemorrhoids, diverticulitis, colon cancer, and varicose veins. When adding insoluble fiber to your diet, remember to drink plenty of fluid so that it can do its softening job.

Soluble fiber has magnet and sponge traits similar to those of insoluble fiber. The difference is that soluble fiber such as oat bran attracts and absorbs cholesterol, which helps prevent heart and gallbladder disease. Soluble fiber also slows glucose absorption from the small intestine, preventing blood sugar fluctuations. The best way to get enough soluble fiber is to eat a variety of whole grains, fruits, and vegetables. Too much fiber can exacerbate GI problems, so again, if you increase the fiber in your diet, do so gradually.

Cholesterol

You mostly hear how bad it is, but cholesterol provides the starting material for the synthesis of sex hormones, adrenal hormones, vitamin D, and bile. The liver makes cholesterol, and there is no need for additional dietary sources. In excess, cholesterol deposits itself on the walls of the arteries, which can interfere with blood flow. Cholesterol is found in food products that come from animals, such as meat, fish, poultry, eggs, and dairy products. It is recommended that less than 300 milligrams be consumed per day.

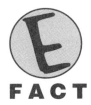

FACT

Lots of foods have cholesterol. For example: one cup of cheddar cheese has 119 mg, one egg has 212 mg, 3/4 cup of coffee has 24 mg, 1 medium ground-beef patty has 74 mg, and one cup of ice cream has 25–145 mg.

A blood profile will report total cholesterol, with numbers also given for *HDL* and *LDL* cholesterol. These are cholesterol designations that refer to the type of protein carriers involved in the transport of cholesterol in blood.

HDL: High Density Lipoprotein (The Good Guys)

HDL collects cholesterol residues and transports them to the liver for reprocessing and excretion. High levels of HDL work to keep the arteries clear of deposits and reduce the risk of coronary artery disease. The best way to elevate HDL cholesterol is through exercise; some research suggests that reducing body fat will also elevate HDL.

LDL: Low Density Lipoprotein (The Bad Guys)

LDL brings cholesterol into the bloodstream to be used for cell building, but it can leave residues of cholesterol on artery walls. Eating foods high in saturated fat stimulates the liver to produce cholesterol, so reducing saturated fat intake is as important as reducing dietary cholesterol.

Blood Glucose and Energy

In addition to the *types* of fuel you put into your body, your energy can be directly linked to the *amount* of energy you put (or don't put) into your body, and the *timing* of it. Nutrition is about fueling the body for optimum function. Many Americans have become so preoccupied with weight loss that they have lost sight of the main event: you need food and the energy source in it—glucose—to live.

If you don't give your body glucose through balanced meals, the brain sends messages that make you feel dizzy and weak. You may also feel irritable, get a headache, and have difficulty concentrating.

If you are not careful when you are hungry, you will eat anything around just to feed yourself because it's as if your brain thinks it's starving. This is why we end up craving high-sugar foods.

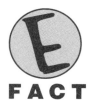

FACT

Most high-sugar foods are also high-fat foods, which packs a double caloric whammy. In fact, nutritionists have postulated that we are as addicted to fat as we are to sugar. This is why balanced, well-timed meals prevent weight gain: you are less likely to reach for non-nutritious foods because you don't get hungry as often.

When you eat quickly, you override the built-in "I'm full" mechanism that the stomach sends out to the brain. This causes you to overeat, and to feel overfull and, sometimes, ill. You also have taken in more energy (calories) than your body needs. Then in frustration, you chastise yourself: "Why did I do that?" So, you proclaim, "Okay, I'll skip the next meal to make up for it." When you try to skip meals, you end up feeling so hungry you tend to overeat all over again. This cycle is physically undesirable and emotionally draining. But you can avoid it.

Two Effective Fitness Eating Plans

Only a licensed nutritionist can truly give someone a personalized eating plan that will work for them. However, there are some general rules to eating well that will keep your energy up. Following are three eating plans that focus on building muscle, decreasing body fat, and maintaining caloric balance so that your workouts won't leave you tired, but instead will contribute to your feeling balanced and energetic.

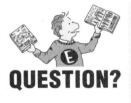

QUESTION?

What are antioxidants, and how do they help my body?
Antioxidants are compounds that protect the body from oxidation or "rust," i.e., what we used to think of as the physical aging process. Antioxidant-rich foods include broccoli, cauliflower, kale, dark chocolate, tea, dark green leafy vegetables, and citrus fruits, many of which include Vitamins E and A, as well as the minerals selenium, and, in chocolate's case, stearic acid. A balanced diet ensures that you'll get a wide variety of antioxidants.

As anyone who has walked into a bookstore knows, there is a recommended eating plan for every separate person on the planet, and then some. And each plan contradicts the other: Eat six meals! Eat five meals, and don't eat after six! Eat no white foods! Eat foods of all colors! Eat mostly protein! Eat mostly carbs! The point is, like exercise, the way you eat is very personal. You will have to figure out what works best for you. Some people need to eat after dinner, or else food is all they think about in the evenings. Some people hate breakfast (even though everyone says you should have it). Some people have to have desserts, while others go off on a binge if they have a bit of chocolate. There is no one right way to eat except for two rules:

- Eat as much as you need to, but no more and no less.
- Eat whole foods, not processed stuff.

Eating Plan #1

This eating plan focuses on eating six small meals throughout the day. Whenever there is no beverage listed, you should drink water with the meal. Now many trainers and nutritionists recommend eating this way because it keeps your blood sugar steady. This is also good for people who like to eat, as you go only a couple of hours between meals.

Day one

Breakfast: 1 hard-boiled egg, 1 orange, ½ cup oatmeal, coffee or tea

Snack: Glass of V8 juice, three whole-wheat crackers with one ounce of hard cheese

Lunch: Salad with grilled shrimp, oil and vinegar

Snack: Small handful of almonds, apple

Dinner: 3 ounces broiled salmon, broccoli and cauliflower, ½ cup brown rice

Snack: 2 butter cookies, glass of milk

Day two

Breakfast: Whole-wheat toast with peanut butter, banana

Snack: Cappuccino with skim milk, 1 biscotti

Lunch: Minestrone soup with 2 tablespoons parmesan cheese

Snack: Baked chips with salsa

Dinner: 3 ounces steak with fat trimmed off, baked potato, peas and carrots

Snack: ½ cup cereal, ½ cup low-fat milk

Day Three

Breakfast: Breakfast burrito

Snack: Orange with 1 ounce low-fat mozzarella

Lunch: Turkey with lettuce and tomato on whole-wheat bread, apple

Snack: Six-ounce mixed berry smoothie made with low-fat yogurt

Dinner: Stir-fried vegetables with shrimp

Snack: ½ cup chocolate ice cream

This plan requires that each meal and snack be relatively small, because if you're eating six times throughout the day but don't want to overeat, you have to be careful about the calorie count of each meal.

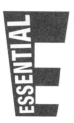

Wine with dinner? Yes! Alcohol (even small amounts of liquor) does have a place in a healthy diet. Just remember: a serving is four ounces of wine (less than half a glass), and most of us drink six to eight ounces at a time. Sip slowly, because alcohol has been shown to reduce the amount of fat the body burns.

Eating Plan #2

For some people, eating three meals and three snacks each day is actually inconvenient and unappetizing. You might be someone who enjoys sitting down to a proper meal, and find snacks unnecessary. This is fine. You just need to make sure your meals are well balanced and that you don't let too much time pass between each meal.

Day One

Breakfast: 1 cup oatmeal made with skim milk, blueberries, two scrambled eggs. Coffee or tea.

Lunch: Tuna on lettuce with tomatoes and peppers, one slice whole-grain bread, sliced apple.

Dinner: Lean steak, baked potato, green beans with almonds. 1 glass red wine. Slice of chocolate cake.

Day Two

Breakfast: Whole-grain flax waffles, strawberries, maple syrup. Link sausages. Coffee or tea.

Lunch: All-natural peanut butter on whole-grain bread, a banana, a small square of dark chocolate. Glass of milk or iced tea.

Dinner: Poached salmon with spinach and wild rice, salad. Dark beer. Sorbet.

Day Three

Breakfast: Omelet with peppers and onions. Coffee or tea.

Lunch: Fruit salad with cottage cheese. Iced tea.

Dinner: Salad. Coq au vin with mashed potatoes. Apple tart.

If you eat this way, you should feel free to have dessert after dinner, and maybe some fruit with breakfast and lunch. If you're used to snacking in between meals, you might feel hungry at those times, but remember, without snacks you can eat a little more at each meal.

Chapter 18
Supplements

Multivitamins. Fat burners. Women's formulas. Calcium-magnesium-zinc combinations. The supplement shelves of your grocery store, drug store, and natural-health store are stocked with little bottles filled with pills. The problem is that most consumers know very little about supplements and are easily swayed by the pills that promise results (weight loss, more energy) but these consumers don't necessarily understand which supplements they may actually need. Supplements can really help make up for a diet lacking in specific nutrients.

What Are Supplements?

In the Dietary Supplement Health and Education Act (DSHEA) of 1994, Congress defined the term "dietary supplement" as a product taken by mouth that contains a "dietary ingredient" intended to supplement the diet. The "dietary ingredients" in these products may include vitamins, minerals, herbs or other botanicals, amino acids, and substances such as enzymes, organ tissues, glandulars, and metabolites.

Dietary supplements can also be extracts or concentrates, and may be found in many forms, such as tablets, capsules, softgels, gelcaps, liquids, or powders. They can also be in other forms, such as a bar, but if they are, information on their label must not represent the product as a conventional food or a the sole item of a meal or diet. DSHEA places dietary supplements (whatever their form may be) in a special category under the general umbrella of foods, not drugs, and requires that every supplement be labeled as such.

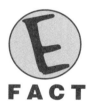

FACT

Some supplements are helpful and can help you if you need to skip a meal or if you have a nutritional shortfall in your diet. Read the labels to be sure you're getting the caloric amount you need to feel full, as well as a balanced amount of nutrients. If you can, add some real food (like yogurt or an apple) to the supplement for more satisfaction.

One issue that comes up with supplements is that people will often try to use them as alternatives to meals. The first immediate issue, obviously, is that we all know the difference between a protein bar and a multivitamin. One provides calories and can be a meal; the other provides very, very few calories and can't be construed as food. The Food and Drug Administration (FDA) regulates dietary supplements under a different set of regulations than those covering conventional foods and drug products. Under the DSHEA of 1994, the dietary supplement manufacturer is responsible for ensuring that a dietary supplement is safe before it is marketed. The FDA is responsible for taking action against any unsafe dietary supplement product after it reaches the market. Generally, manufacturers do not need to register their products with the FDA nor get FDA approval before producing or selling dietary supplements. Manufacturers must make sure that product label information is truthful and not misleading.

Doctor-recommended Supplements

Most doctors, personal trainers, fitness teachers, and nutritionists take supplements. Some take a pile of pills a day, while others just take a multivitamin to make up for anything their diet might lack. Some take vitamin E to ward off heart disease, while others take calcium for bone loss, or folic acid to prevent birth defects.

Most experts agree—although no groups officially recommend—that you take a multivitamin supplement (that includes some minerals, too) for general health insurance. These supplements will rarely give you too much of a certain vitamin, while they may ensure that you actually get enough of what you need.

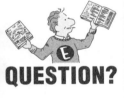

QUESTION?

Can I get my vitamins and minerals from fortified cereal?
Yes. The only problem with many fortified cereals is that they contain a high amount of processed flour and sugar, which aren't good for you. If your choice is between a bowl of corn flakes and whole milk, or two slices of whole-wheat bread with peanut butter plus a multivitamin, eat the more nutritious food and take the supplement. The calories are being delivered in a much healthier way via the bread and peanut butter, including more fiber, less sugar, and healthy fats and protein.

You might consider an antioxidant supplement, such as vitamins C and E, especially if you don't eat a lot of fruits and vegetables. Other specific recommendations are for B vitamins (good for mood regulation and the reproductive system, especially if you're a vegetarian), and a calcium-magnesium-zinc supplement if you fear bone loss, or don't consume dairy products.

Supplements Doctors Don't Recommend

The government controls—pretty tightly—what a supplement can claim and not claim on its labels. However, as you well know, numerous little bottles make promises, such as "Burn more energy!" or "Lose more weight!" Of course, you are rarely told what is in these bottles, so it's hard to know what research, if any, is behind these claims. And by the time the government gets around to getting the ineffective pills off the shelves, they have already sold millions of dollars' worth of product (in the best case) or have hurt or killed people (in the worst case).

In general, stay away from any supplement that makes grand promises. Most multivitamin and mineral supplements don't promise anything. They simply tell you what they're designed to do, such as aid women's bodies or provide the nutrients a vegetarian diet might be lacking. Those are explanations, not promises.

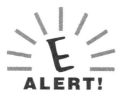

ALERT!

Just because supplements are sold over the counter doesn't mean they don't interact with medicines or other supplements. They do, so before you take something, do some research and talk to your doctor or a nutritionist about whether a specific supplement is right for you and your particular health situation.

Now, having said that, some nutrients that aren't vitamins and minerals, such as herbs, protein supplements, and certain fats, are helpful to you. Some possibilities that you might want to investigate are whey and other proteins to build muscle and help promote weight loss; DHEA and fish oils to aid brain function and reduce inflammation throughout the body; and certain herbs for moods, joint problems, and pain reduction.

Caffeine

One of the world's most popular drugs, caffeine is a stimulant that affects the central nervous system, the digestive tract, and the metabolism. Caffeine is found in coffee beans, tea leaves, cocoa beans, and products derived from these sources. It is absorbed quickly in the body and can raise blood pressure, the heart rate, and brain serotonin levels (low levels of serotonin cause drowsiness). Withdrawal from caffeine can cause headaches and drowsiness. The pharmacological active dose of caffeine is defined as 200 milligrams, and the daily recommended not-to-exceed intake level is the equivalent of one to three cups of coffee per day (139 to 417 milligrams).

You get caffeine—and more than you think—in numerous ways. A brewed cup of coffee has about 139 mg of caffeine, a brewed cup of tea (not herbal) has 48 mg of caffeine, one cup of semisweet chocolate chips has 92 mg, and one ounce of bittersweet chocolate has 18–30 mg. If you feel nervous or jittery, try to find a balance between how much caffeine helps you focus, and how much leaves you on edge.

Sports Drinks

Lots of people (many of whom aren't burning that many calories) think sports drinks, such as Gatorade and other energy replenishers, are more nutritious than water. This is not true. While these drinks have their place in a real endurance athlete's life, people who are simply working out do not need the extra calories (from sugar) that give these drinks their flavor and energy. In fact, most nutritionists consider sports drinks to be no healthier than soda. And soda has no nutritional value at all.

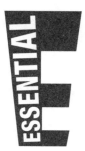

The added sugar in sports drinks is not only bad for your waistline, but also hurts your teeth, too. If you do reach for these drinks every once in a while, be sure to at least rinse with water afterward to keep the sugar from hurting your enamel.

Even those bottled waters with additives that aren't sugar (such as teas or minerals) that claim to boost your mood or reduce fat are only marketing ploys. None of these bottled waters have been shown to effectively fulfill their claims.

Make Your Own Sports Drink

If you do need to add some flavor to your water, try putting fruit in (orange is delicious, but you can even add watermelon or strawberries). Lots of spas offer their clients water with cucumber slices, which is highly refreshing.

You can also use fruit teas for flavor or, if you want, mix some juice with water to create a flavor you like. Some good additions to water include straight cranberry juice (not cocktail) with lime (it's like a virgin Cosmopolitan) or orange juice with a little cherry juice for a virgin Tequila Sunrise.

Stay Away from Anything Fizzy

Bubbles have no place in your belly when you're exercising, as they will create gas, which can lead to cramps and discomfort. Even drinking carbonated liquids after you exercise isn't good for you, as it creates a sense of fullness (that you can see if you look down at your torso) that takes away from the natural diuretic effect of exercise.

If you love the refreshing taste of bubbly water, save it for a few hours after you exercise, or have it with a meal. But try to sip it slowly to reduce the gas effect.

Meal Replacements

You're hungry, but you don't have time for a full lunch. Or perhaps you've heard about the success of diets in which two meals a day are either shakes or bars, and the third meal is a regular one. Or maybe you know weightlifters and personal trainers who swear by protein bars and other supplements. Do meal-replacement supplements work?

The answer is yes, but there are some issues about using them. The good thing about meal replacements, whether they are bars or shakes, is that they do usually provide a good amount of nutrients for the calorie count. So for example, if your choice is between chips, cookies, and another snack food, or having a meal-replacement supplement, go for the meal replacement. It's more nutritious and will probably be more filling.

Also, because the replacement foods are properly balanced in terms of nutrients and calories, you could ostensibly lose weight by eating them if you're replacing high-fat, high-calorie foods in your diet with the meal-replacement bars or shakes. As long as you supplement them with real, whole food, there is a good chance you'll not only lose weight but also feel good and stay healthy.

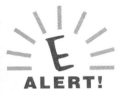

ALERT!

Feel free to rely on meal-replacement foods sometimes, but remember, no bar or shake tastes as good as the right portions of steak, salad, a baked potato, and a glass of wine. Meal-replacement foods are useful only if they are substituted for unhealthy foods, not nutritious, satisfying meals.

There are, however, some negative issues with meal replacements. The first is that there are numerous nutrients in food, such as antioxidants, that are not included in supplements, so even if supplements are nutritious, they aren't whole foods. Second, not all protein and meal-replacement bars and shakes are created equal. Some are high in fat, some are high in sugar, and some just don't have the nutrients they claim to have. It's difficult to distinguish one from the other.

Read the Label

If you do need to use a meal-replacement shake or bar, look for those that have between 200 and 400 calories, with at least 25 percent of those calories coming from protein. It should also include at least 23 vitamins and minerals (which is more than most foods have). It's also helpful if the meal replacement has at least five or six grams of fiber.

Don't be afraid to complement these food substitutes with real food. These calorie amounts aren't that high, so it's perfectly acceptable to add a piece of fruit or some raw vegetables (and hummus, too!) to round out your meal.

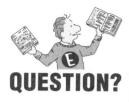

QUESTION?

I lost weight with shakes, and now I'm afraid to eat real food.
It's understandable to be nervous, but remember that you lost weight not because of the meal replacements, but because you decreased how many calories you ate and increased how much you moved. As long as your intake and output are in balance, you will maintain your healthy weight. Remember, you can always go back to shakes if the real foods aren't easy enough for you to control.

One of the biggest problems with meal replacements is that they don't give diners the emotional and mental satisfaction that a real meal provides. So if you're eating a meal replacment, try to be sure that your next meal is a real one. Sit down at a table, and eat slowly rather than rushing, so that you feel satisfied on all levels.

Stay Away from Added Ingredients

When you read the labels on meal replacements, look for ingredients that are actual food (nuts and whey, for example), and stay away from ingredients that claim to improve health on their own. Herbal supplements, carbohydrate blockers, or too much protein aren't going to make you healthier or fitter.

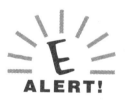

ALERT!

If you can only reach for a candy bar as a meal, make it a Snickers. The nuts and calories will fill you up, so you will probably not need to eat more than the candy bar itself. Just make sure your next meal is a healthy one and includes salad or vegetables, as well as a source of protein that has little or no saturated fat. This will balance out the candy bar in your daily diet.

If the bar or shake has sugar or corn syrup as one of its first few ingredients, then it is no more than a candy bar. Also, look at the nutrition label to see what percentage of the bar is added sugar or saturated fats. Those are both unhealthy ingredients and won't help you be healthy or keep your weight in check.

Chapter 19

Easy Fitness for Kids

Until just a few years ago, kids were the best example adults had for what an active, fit life should look like. Unfortunately, between video games, long rides (rather than walks) to school, and slashes in school budgets for gym and athletics, kids have become the new face—or body—for the growing obesity problem. In this chapter, you'll learn why it's so important for kids to stay active these days, as well as ways to help kids keep moving.

Activity Is Natural

They can't wait to crawl and then walk and then run. They want to play catch even when they don't know how, and they want to play sports even when they don't understand the concepts of teamwork and competition. Kids are proof that we come into this world wanting to move and be active. It is the rare child who can—or wants to—sit still.

It's a shame, then, that adults believe that kids need to learn how to sit still. Sitting still is certainly not what our bodies were meant to do. More than that, the whole sit-still way of thinking is part of what creates sedentary adults. Even more dangerous, this mentality is creating a generation of overweight kids.

There is no stronger proof of what the current Western way of life is doing to people than the shape of our children, because kids are naturally active. Kids still love to move and play.

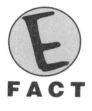

FACT

If you watch children play, you'll notice that they do intervals! They run around really fast for a few minutes, then fall over onto the grass and lie there for a few seconds to recover. They race around the pool, then do nothing. They jump and run and shout and skip, then sit and drink some lemonade. Kids don't count calories or worry about their heart rate or wonder if their workout is too much. They just go and go and go until they can't go anymore, and then they stop.

Kids also make a game out of everything. If they walk across the street, they skip or try to hop over the grate. If they see a lamppost, they'll race you to it. Children find movement to be not only fun but also natural. In other words, it is in their nature to move, and when they listen to their bodies, they move as much as they need to.

Are Computers and TVs the Enemies?

It is not that computers or TV are inherently bad, and the point of this section isn't to argue that kids shouldn't watch *Sesame Street* or do research on the Web. The important thing to know about kids and the computer and TV is that there is a clear line between how much kids watch TV and their weight. Just as with adults, the more sedentary a child is, the more out of shape they will be.

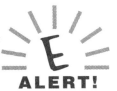

ALERT!

Besides the immediate health risks, kids who are overweight will have a harder time staying healthy as they grow older. Every part of their body will be affected, from their mood to their growth and their heart to their reproductive systems. It is harder for adults who were heavy as children to lose weight, and it is more likely that fat children will carry obesity-related illnesses with them into adulthood.

It is often difficult, as a parent, to set boundaries about TV and the computer, but it is easier if you set a good example. If your child's TV needs to be off, shut yours off, too. If you want her to take more walks, go with her. Studies have shown that teenagers these days do not necessarily look at their parents as objects they should rebel against; many teenagers admire and want to spend time with their parents. Use that fact as your own inspiration to get out and be more active. It will help both of you.

Embarrassment about Weight

Fat camps. Weigh-ins. The stares. It's awful for kids to be overweight, even though it's more and more common. A child is no more responsible for her weight than she is for her way of life or for her choice of foods. Kids move as much as they re given the opportunity to.

Of course, some children's genetics predispose them to weight problems, and if you are a family member, you probably struggle with those issues, too. The most important thing you can do as a parent is simply offer your children as many healthy and nutritious foods as possible. Also, if they want to eat a fun snack or treat, let them, being sure to control the amount they eat, as well as making sure that the "treat" isn't too unhealthy. For example, a small piece of chocolate is better than a highly processed fruit snack.

Withholding the foods other kids eat will only make them want it more, and at the same time, not teach them how to eat proper servings as well as how to deal with their cravings.

Also, teach your kids about their bodies. Don't assume that because they are kids they can't handle nutritional information. Teach them about servings, nutrients, calories, and exercise. Let them know what they can control about their weight and what they can't. In other words, explain that exercise and food can contribute to their weight, but that they can't be taller or change their shape very dramatically.

While this should go without saying, remember that no one—adult or child—has ever lost weight and kept it off because they have been humiliated or because someone else controlled their food intake. In fact, studies have shown that children whose parents curtail their diets grow up to be overweight. It is far better to have a child respond to his or her own hunger—if they are kept active and engaged in activities—than to worry about dieting and weight.

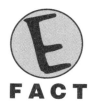

FACT

Whatever the specific image problem or weight issue (real or imagined), there are three "people" involved in a child's body image problem or eating disorder: society—which values thinness but promotes obesity; you—because chances are you struggle yourself with food and image; and your child—who is suffering from a problem that can become very serious.

These days, both boys and girls suffer from body image problems and eating disorders. Girls perceive themselves to be fat and do anything to be thin, while boys can have the problem of either being skinny and wanting to be muscular, or want to be thinner because they think they need to lose a few pounds.

Here are some signs that your child has an eating disorder: preoccupation with weight, food, calories, and dieting; exercise is excessive and rigid even if your child is fatigued, ill, hurt, or the weather is very bad; your child constantly complains about being fat even though she is at a normal weight; your child compares her body to others; evidence of vomiting, such as smells in the bathroom; your child disappears after meals; your child uses laxatives, diuretics, diet pills, or enemas; your child seems to consume large amounts of food but doesn't gain weight; your child hoards food; fluctuating weight; cessation or erratic menstrual cycles; obsession with appearance as a definition of self and perfectionist thinking; refusal to eat meals with family; food rituals, such as eating a very limited variety of foods and cutting food into small pieces.

If you suspect your child has an eating disorder or is using steroids or other supplements to build muscle or gain or lose weight, maintain clear, kind and decisive communication without blaming, anger, or pity. Talk to your child about her life without focusing on food; expect your child to eat with your family (you eat together, right?), but don't demand that she eat; be physically affectionate and loving. Don't demand that your child gain weight, and don't blame the child and tell her she is responsible for family problems or your problems. Don't allow her eating problem to dominate the family's eating schedule. Get her into therapy and under a doctor's care and then let her work the problem out with your support, not under your control.

Changing Kids' Lifestyles

Of course, it isn't easy to change another person's habits, even a kid's, but there are right ways to help a child and wrong ways to "try" to help. The first thing is to realize that if kids have lived sedentary lives, then they need to be taught how to live an active life. So invite them to do something fun, like ice skating or going for a walk around a park. Rather than talk about their weight, talk about the rewards of being active, including how good it feels and how much fun it will be to buy clothes. Do not talk about the health benefits of weight loss or fitness because most kids feel invincible. However, if the child has an illness like diabetes you should talk to them about how much their lives will improve with exercise.

If you feel like you aren't helping your child, consider joining a gym and finding a personal trainer or coach who knows what she is doing and is supportive and accepting rather than tough. Tough love does not help a child develop a lifelong relationship with fitness.

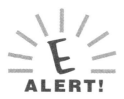

ALERT!

Do not push a child to do more than she is able. If she is overweight, don't force her to run or bike for longer than she can. The most important thing is that you are loving and encouraging. Reward activity, not weight loss. Help a child find a sport or activity she likes and wants to become better at, rather than expecting them to "exercise," because kids need something that engages them and helps them feel good about themselves.

Of course, inactivity isn't the only problem when it comes to child obesity. Food is also a major issue. If you have a kid who eats vegetables and fruit, and shuns most sugary things, consider yourself lucky—and rare. If not, here are a few things you can do.

First, control breakfast. Some cereals—those with whole grains—are healthy; others—the ones with lots of sugar—aren't. Children who eat a good breakfast not only have better health, they also do better in school (because they aren't tired and their bodies are functioning optimally). Be sure your child's breakfast includes a low-fat protein, a whole grain, and fruits or vegetables. For example, breakfast could be berries in cereal or salsa on eggs.

Reduce the damage lunch can do. Most school lunches are non-nutritious and fattening. If your child wants to buy her lunch, at least read the menu in advance and help her make good choices. Ask her to get a salad, or have an apple to go with the fries. Adding healthy foods is easier to do than refusing unhealthy foods.

With snacks, let your child mix it up between unhealthy and healthy. Rather than riding her about "bad" choices, be sure she has some "good" choices at home; apples with peanut butter, crackers and cheese, salsa and baked chips are all nutritious options.

Eat dinner with your child. This is really one of the most important things you can do with your child, not only for her health but also for her well-being. Once again, focus on low-fat protein, whole grains, and fresh vegetable side dishes. Dessert? Absolutely. Show her that you, too, can enjoy good food in moderation.

Fun Games and Activities

What is fun activity for a two-year-old is ridiculous for a nine-year-old. Following are some ideas for age-appropriate games and activities for kids. Of course, some activities are ageless: walking, biking, swimming, hiking, and dancing can be done by every member of the family. Granted, young children will need to be in strollers or carried, but that doesn't mean they won't benefit from being included in the activity, because seeing you being active will encourage them to move when they get older.

Up to Three Years Old

Get out your exercise ball and hold your baby or toddler on it. Let them roll around while they sit or lie down on it; just keep a good grip on them. Even though they won't be conscious of it, this kind of playing will improve their balance. You can also do things like this on skateboards and other gym tools that improve balance. Just remember: they can't do this on their own; you need to hold onto them.

Turn on the radio or your favorite CD, and hold your child in your arms, and dance. Vary the tempo and your steps. Let them feel your body move, and sing to them, too.

Go to the playground and the beach. If it's cold, bundle your kids up and get outside even if it's just for a few minutes. And get on the slides and jungle gym with your kids, it's good for them to see you moving.

Three to Five Years Old

Kids this age will love to do what you're doing. So stand up and stomp your feet, clap your hands, skip, hop, dance, whatever; then ask them to follow the leader. Make sure they get a turn as leader, too.

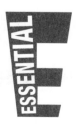

Don't go expect too much from young children who are learning about sports because your competitive edge will make the experience stressful for them. Instead, encourage them to enjoy moving rather than improving any skills that are necessary for the game.

This is a good age for kids to start learning sports-related activities, like batting, throwing, catching, kicking, and running. Focus on specific skills, such as keeping your eye on the ball, using both feet rather than your hands, or aiming. Be sure the equipment is age appropriate, too, including smaller balls and props, such as batting tees.

Make sure you are encouraging, and understand that young bodies do not have the control or strength that grade-school children have. Also, kids this age aren't yet ready for lots of team activities, as it is hard for them to wait and understand rules.

Early School Age

Now is the time to bring your sons and daughters to team sports and activities that focus on cooperation and skills, not winning (don't worry, we'll get to winning in a few years). Right now, they need to learn how to wait, how to take their turn, and then how to do what they need to when they're up to bat, on defense, or have the ball.

Try many different things: ice skating, gymnastics, horseback riding, ballet, dancing, karate, fencing, Ping-Pong, bowling, sledding, rollerblading, water skiing, swimming, diving. You just never know what your child will enjoy and be good at. And let them see you try new activities, too, even if you aren't good at them. In fact, it's an especially good lesson for them to see you struggle and practice to learn a new skill—and keep a smile on your face the whole time.

Older School Age

At this age, your child probably has a sport he enjoys—and is good at—more than others. Rather than focusing on the competition, you should help children refine their skills and study what makes the better players do so well. Let them see that excelling at a sport involves both talent and practice. Encourage your child to study both amateur and professional players and learn strategies about the game or sport they like. Even now, though, don't focus on winning as much as you focus on skills and practice.

Remember to have fun. Once a child picks a sport or skill she enjoys, she needs to remember that being active is a way to enjoy herself, not just win. So be sure they get outside for walks and for activities, such as touch football on Sundays and swimming during the summer. Especially since kids get self-conscious, you want to be sure they feel confident about their bodies (no matter what their bodies look like).

Active Girls

While an involvement in sports helps both boys and girls, girls benefit in very specific ways from joining teams and having a strong commitment to a physical activity. For example, high-school female athletes are less likely to smoke than nonathletes. And a 1998 study definitively linked sports involvement and lowered rates of teenage pregnancy.

Following are more benefits that girls enjoy from sports:

- Girls involved in high-school sports have higher science grades and test scores. They are less likely to drop out of high school and more likely to go on to college than their nonathletic counterparts.
- Girls who engage in regular physical activity are less likely to be overweight. They have lower levels of blood sugar, cholesterol and tryglycerides, and lower blood pressure than nonexercising girls.
- Girls who participate in sports teams feel better about their bodies than those who don't.

The good effects last for years. Girls who exercise develop stronger, denser bones, and are less likely to develop osteoporosis. Also, even small amounts of exercise per week can reduce the risk of breast cancer in later life. Sports can help in other areas of life—80 percent of female Fortune 500 executives described themselves as "tomboys" and were involved in athletics when they were young.

Group Sports

The dropout rate of kids from group sports is around 70 percent, according to some research. The reasons? Parents, and bad coaching. Kids used to just play sports with their friends for fun, not necessarily for future scholarships or the ability to make their parents proud.

If you're committed to keeping your child active and you recognize the benefit group sports provide for kids, then you need to be very involved in your child's team. Your involvement is important because most group sports need levelheaded parents to provide support and leadership to the kids.

Level-headedness is important, because many parents who care more about winning try to take over kids' teams, which leaves many of the children feeling discouraged. Instead, help your children and their teammates focus on skills and good sportsmanship. This isn't to say that winning doesn't matter.

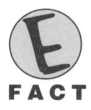

FACT

Children will not gain the benefits of the important lessons team sports offer if a thoughtful and communicative adult isn't around to discuss the experience with them. After a game, be sure to talk with your child about how the game went and how they felt about it. Remind them that playing well and that improving skills are more important than winning.

For children, competing doesn't have to be about winning. You can encourage your child and his team to focus on playing their best. Understanding the ups and downs of team sports helps kids develop good emotional intelligence, not just physical skills.

In the real world, of course, competitiveness is useful—it helps you improve yourself, get jobs, study harder, and practice when you aren't doing as well as you would like. It's a measure of success. What you need to remember is that winning is important, but that most winners get the point of both the game and the skills before they become winners. In other words, winning is more likely to come as a result of practice, not as a result of a competitive, mean-spirited attitude.

Active Kids Benefit You, Too!

If you're struggling with fitness, one of the best things to do is spend some time with kids. You'll notice that they move far more than you do. But if you can, it's good to try to keep up with them. They're going to exhaust you, but don't let yourself blame your age for your lethargy. The difference in your energy level isn't all about age, but about socialization.

"Sit down!" "Sit still!" "Can't you just be quiet!" All of these things that we say to our children, we say when we want peace and quiet, or when we ourselves want to rest. But it is often in those moments when it would be good for adults to be active and use that time to exercise their bodies.

And yet, adults often expect children to walk at the same pace they do or to move as quickly as they do. Whether it's putting on their coats or taking a walk, when kids want to take their time, they do.

And that too, is a natural form of body wisdom, because bodies, as you've learned, also need time to use low amounts of energy. So a walk down the block that takes a half hour because of how interesting all the weeds look peeking through the sidewalk cracks? That's natural, too.

So, if you can spend a day or two with some young kids (without a TV nearby, of course), try to keep up with them and, at the same time, try to slow down with them. See how you feel at the end of the day. Chances are you'll feel energized and yet tired. Children, if they haven't yet been overly socialized, move as much as they need to, and when they are given the opportunity, they take great care of their bodies.

Chapter 20

Easy Fitness for Seniors

As we age, the simple tasks we always took for granted become more challenging. Suddenly it's impossible to open a jar of spaghetti sauce, and dancing with your husband is more of a chore than a fun activity. If ever there was a reason to stay fit, it's for the quality of life you can maintain and even improve when you are older. This chapter explains the way the body changes as it ages, and offers some great tips for physical and mental workouts for seniors.

20

Balance Issues

Falling scares people. It scares them psychologically because falling could cause them to break their bones, or cause another injury from which they wouldn't recover completely. As people age, many of them (mostly those who haven't been exercising regularly) start to feel less confident about their ability to do everyday things, such as walk and take care of their homes.

Their fear, unfortunately, is not unfounded. As they age, many people lose primary and secondary physical skills, which makes navigating everyday life a challenge. For example, if your peripheral vision has diminished it might be difficult to continue dancing or going running. If your memory is compromised, you might find following the directions in an exercise class confusing. If your muscles are weak and your flexibility has decreased, then even walking a short distance might be hard for your legs. And if you've lost your sense of balance and agility, if you slip you might be unable to recover, and you might fall.

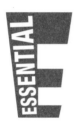

Regular exercise, even if it's begun at a very advanced age, has been shown to help stave off heart disease, type 2 diabetes, and other serious diseases; help maintain brain health and function; it also maintains and can even improve bone density. It also offers an opportunity for socializing and decreases the likelihood of the onset of age-related depression and anxiety.

Once you've fallen, if your health is not what it used to be, your body will find it harder to recover. And if you're afraid—of losing your independence, of being sick and dependent, of falling again—then your fear might change your mood and demeanor.

But it doesn't have to be this way. You've learned that aging can be just about numbers, not about a decline in ability. When it comes to balance, you only need to know two things: balance is a function of your brain's ability to sense your body's place in space, and your sense of balance is the result of practice that your body has done in regaining its balance over and over again throughout life.

For example, when you step onto an escalator, you regain your balance. When you ride a bike, you are maintaining your balance without the use of your feet. When you reach up to get something out of a cabinet and stand on one foot, you are using your balance.

The truth is, balance is an always-fluctuating ability. For example, you can get up from a chair and find it easy to stand up straight, you start to walk and that's easy, and you continue to walk up a hill and you're doing fine. But suddenly, there's a little rock under your foot that you didn't see, and your foot slips . . . and you find it impossible to regain your balance and you fall.

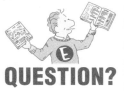

QUESTION?

What is the best way to improve balance?
Practice yoga or tai chi. Both require you to stand on one foot and shift your weight from one foot to the other at various times throughout the routines. Also, these practices ask that you get comfortable with the possibility of falling. This may sound odd, but balance is less about being still and more about being as steady as possible. As a living organism, the body is never completely still. Instead, you need to be always steadying yourself as you move, which is exactly what you do when you practice yoga and tai chi.

Balance is always moving and changing, and the skill of balance is one of adjustment. What older people need, when it comes to balance, is not the ability to stand still, but the ability to get hold of themselves when their feet go out from under them. If you stay in shape as you get older, you are less likely to fall, but if you do fall, you are less likely to get injured and, if you do get injured, you are more likely to heal faster and with fewer repercussions.

Resistance to Activity

For decades, society held two general attitudes toward exercise. First, people believed that it wasn't ladylike. Second, many thought that it was a kind of mindless, low-life activity. White-collar jobs were seen as the gateway to a higher quality way of life, and activities where you would sweat or get dirty were less than appealing.

Because these attitudes were considered correct for so long, it's difficult, sometimes, to get older people to want to exercise or to be open to the benefits of activity. This is especially true when activity seems to exacerbate health problems. For example, when someone older or out of shape starts an exercise program or attempts to be active, they may experience some aches and pains from the changes. This discomfort will often make the person want to stop their new program. Even when you tell this person that activity will, in the long run, make them happier and healthier, they might only recognize that activity is making them feel tired and achy. On top of this, because the idea of exercise as beneficial is a new one, it's difficult to teach seniors what you know about fitness without coming across as, well, a know-it-all kid, no matter what your age.

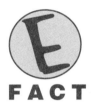

FACT

Need motivation to keep fit? How's this? Older people who exercise regularly experience fewer aches and pains than other people their age who are less active. Researchers found elderly people who engaged in brisk aerobic exercise, like running, had 25 percent less joint and muscle pain.

So, if you love and care for an older person, be respectful of their point of view and recognize that their attitude toward exercise and fitness may not be the same as yours. You might even try telling them about your experience working out and asking them whether they were active when they were young. Before you attempt to offer advice or encouragement, first offer them validation of their opinions.

Encouragement Is the Best Medicine

As with giving advice to anyone else, the first rule of thumb is: Don't point out what seniors are doing wrong, as in "you should exercise more." Any "should" statement is, in general, not that helpful. Instead, the following are some ideas on how to offer encouragement to an older person.

Invite them to be active with you. Even if they walk slower then you walk, or worry about the weather and their doubts that exercise will actually help their health, ask them along on the walk or any other family outing. In other words, invite them to join you, and be both respectful yet challenging. If they shrug off throwing a ball down the lane or walking up the bleachers, be relaxed but explain that you believe activity would help them feel better, and that you'd enjoy sharing the activity with them.

Enlist the advice of their doctor. If your friend or parent doubts that exercise would help his health, accompany them to the doctor and ask the doctor his opinion of exercise. Don't tell the doctor that you think exercise will help (the older person in your life will see this as insulting to the physician). Instead, rely on some humble questions so it seems as if the advice comes from the doctor, not you.

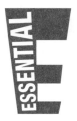

Think gentle and easy. Swimming, walking, and ballroom dancing are all activities that might appeal to an older person. If you love the gym, don't assume that your parent will, too. Instead, find out if there is any activity they like or have always wanted to do, or ask what might appeal to them. Let them pick and choose what they'll enjoy, not what you think they should do.

Ask your kids to help out. Sometimes the generation gap actually skips… a generation. Have your kids invite their grandparents along for a walk or activity. This will make your parent feel young and not belittled.

Loneliness, isolation, and boredom are as dangerous to older people as illness. If you know an older person who sits and watches TV most of the day, rest assured that even just a few minutes of interaction and a quiet activity, such as croquet or golf, can make a big difference. Even 10 minutes of activity can make all the difference in someone's health, while a total of 30 minutes of daily exercise can actually mean reaching a good level of fitness.

Also, scientifically speaking, older people don't have to take part in high-intensity activities to see benefits, so don't get into the details of heart rate or a fitness program. Instead, think about activities they'll enjoy.

Mental Fitness

In 2005, Ohio State University researchers reported that older people who exercised regularly were more likely to maintain the mental acuity they needed to do everyday tasks like follow a recipe and keep track of the pills they take. Some of the recommended mental activities for older people included crossword puzzles, trivia games, Scrabble, card games, and projects, such as fixing appliances and cooking.

Rather than getting frustrated with the changes in the speed and mental agility of older people, challenge them to think and help you. Reframing your interactions with the goal of helping the older person feel confident and capable (remember the effectiveness of active intentions) will help her become healthier rather than feeling her age.

Remember, too, that mood disorders are a common, but often undiagnosed, problem in older people. Physical activity as well as relief from boredom can help prevent and cure the symptoms of depression, anxiety, grief, and insomnia that affect one in five older Americans.

Group Fitness for Seniors

Another great way to help older people is to encourage them to take part in group activities, including group fitness classes. While this may seem awkward to them at first, once they meet the other participants, who will most likely be their age, they will probably appreciate the interaction as well as the physical rewards.

Try to remember that fear, insecurity, and lack of confidence strike everyone, so be a friend to someone who has to put himself into a new situation, no matter what their age. Taking a new exercise class or having to acknowledge that you are now doing crossword puzzles for mental fitness, rather than fun, isn't easy for anyone.

Chapter 21

Where Do You Go from Here?

Cardiovascular strength and endurance, muscular strength and endurance, flexibility, walking, swimming, strength training...it's a lot of information that all adds up to one important point: you need to move it, or you'll lose it. And what you lose in muscle, cardiovascular function, and strength will make you put on fat and be more susceptible to illness and a decline in your quality of life. On the other hand, creating your easy fitness life will bring you happiness and a better life.

Recommit Every Day

Every day is a new day. And that means every day you will be faced with reasons to not exercise. To eat too much. To eat something unhealthy. To watch something on TV instead of taking a walk. Every day is a new day where you have to recommit to your active life.

Of course, it's overwhelming to think that committing to fitness is something you have to do every day for the rest of your life, because most of us look at exercise as something we will do to reach a goal. Then, we think we will be able to stop working out and yet still be able to hold on to the results. But the truth is, getting fit and staying fit in this day and age really does require recommitting to exercise and eating well every day.

Being Realistic

As we discussed in Chapter 2, exercise and activity are not things we can easily work into our lives in this day and age. While it's certainly more fun and exciting to think that once we set active intentions, we will always easily reach our goals and live active lives, that is an unrealistic expectation. And having unrealistic expectations does not help us reach and keep our goals.

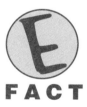

FACT

The number-one reason people give for not exercising is "lack of time." But it's not really about time, but about planning. Even presidents find time to exercise, as do many stay-at-home moms and busy executives. Tom Brokaw is famous for running up and down the stairs in the hotels he stayed in, and Sheryl Crow practiced yoga before her stadium shows. Their secret? Not time, but a place for exercise in their daily schedule.

Therefore, you should plan on surprises and roadblocks. Planning for the obstacles will be your best support in reaching your goals. For example, let's say your number-one goal is to go swimming every Monday, Wednesday, and Friday at the Y. When you write that intention down in your date book (you are doing that, right?), don't delude yourself into thinking that nothing will get in your way. Be honest. Is it a possibility that you're going to have to go to an event at your son's school? Did you remember hearing that your book club might get together on Wednesday rather than Tuesday this month?

Now that you are being honest about and accepting these potential obstructions, you can use that knowledge to work around them. So, continuing our example, figure out what you can do instead of swimming if you have to. Can you take a walk in the morning? Can you swim on Tuesday rather than Wednesday if there is a change in your book club's schedule? Creating alternatives in your schedule will strengthen your resolve and help your reach your goals.

Reversing Backslides

For two weeks you did great. You made every aerobics class, lifted weights every time you said you would, and even managed to stretch for 10 minutes before going to bed every night. But one day a late-night phone call made you skip your stretching, and then a meeting made you miss your aerobics class, and then, suddenly, it's been five days since you exercised.

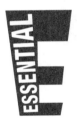

Backslides happen. Be aware that if you can reverse your backslide in less than a week, your fitness level (and weight) won't suffer at all. The truth is, you have two weeks before your body will actually lose what gains it has made with your workouts. Still, it's psychologically difficult to regain momentum once you've lost your rhythm, so the sooner you stop and reverse your backslide, the better.

If you've missed a few days of your workout routine, no worries. Just go back to your date book and pick up where you left off. If, however, you missed a week or more, you might want to take a few days to adjust your routine, making it a little bit easier than usual to give your body a chance to readjust to your program. After a day or two of regular exercise, though, you should be able to go back to the schedule you left.

Finally, if you've missed three weeks to a month of exercise, you might want to start all over again. It won't take as long as it did before to get back to the fitness level you were at, and starting over again will prevent injuries. Here's good news, though: if you've been exercising regularly for a while, there's a very good chance that a short break in your workout schedule will actually improve your fitness level, as rest can make all the difference.

Go Short, Not Long

If you know the next few weeks of your life are going to be busy or stressful or difficult, there is something else you can do to stay fit and healthy. Use 10-minute bursts of exercise to keep your heart in shape, your muscles strong, and your mood uplifted. The best way to do this is, once again, to schedule those workouts. Even though it's only 10 minutes, when you're that busy, those 10 minutes are often hard to find.

In order to make them effective and keep your fitness level where you want it to be, make those 10-minute bursts mean something. Be sure you get cardio, resistance training, and some mind-body routines into your schedule. Once again, be realistic. Don't expect that you will strength train when you aren't near weights, or that you will do yoga in between doctor's appointments. The best time to schedule 10-minute bursts of exercise are when you wake up and before you go to bed.

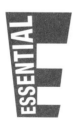

Look at breaks in your routines as opportunities to challenge yourself rather than as inconveniences, and you'll find positive changes will be the result. For example, if your car is in the shop, allow yourself an extra 30 minutes so that you can walk to the grocery store instead of drive. Just wear a backpack so you can carry your groceries home.

Another way to make the bursts of exercise meaningful is to let their intensity level be a bit higher than your usual workout. For example, if you typically walk at a 3.7 mph pace, you might try jogging for 30 seconds two or three times during your 10-minute walks. If you typically strength train with 5-pound dumbbells, use heavier weights, even if it means doing fewer repetitions.

Adapting to Your Lifestyle

Human beings are funny. For instance, as much as we want to lose weight, be toned and fit, and feel more energetic, once we get started the road suddenly seems scary, and we can quickly scurry in the other direction.

Is this fear of success? Lack of commitment? Self-sabotage? Hundreds of books have been written on why so many of us have trouble reaching our goals, and this is not the book for that kind of self-scrutiny. However, because this problem is so widespread, there is a good chance that not only do you recognize it in yourself, but also you can already predict how and when it will happen to you.

So, be honest with yourself about this potential problem, and, once again, as much as possible, be prepared. Take, for example, sleeping late when you want so much to wake up early and walk for 20 minutes. You wake up early and exercise for five days straight. Then one day, you set your alarm clock, and, with seemingly no control the next morning, you hit "snooze," and then spend the majority of your day berating yourself for hitting that button.

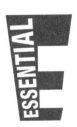

If you are always good for five days, and always get messed up on the sixth, then plan for that sixth day. Know that five days of intention setting and goal reaching is your norm, and adjust your intentions and goals accordingly. For instance, wake up early for five days, take off two days, and then get back on your five-day schedule. Or change your intentions and goals every five days.

Allow for and embrace your personality and quirks. Rather than setting yourself up for what might be considered failure, work with yourself and look at that as success. Success is not sticking to an arbitrary plan (even one that you yourself created), but is, instead, making adjustments every day for long-term health and fitness.

Starting a New Program

A lifetime of fitness relies on you starting new workout programs at regular intervals throughout your life, based on changes in your fitness levels, as well as changes in your life and schedule.

For instance, let's say you've been going along for six months, regularly taking walks in the afternoon and attending yoga classes twice a week. After this amount of time, your body has become used to this program and no longer gets the same fitness kick from the activity that it used to. So if you want to continue to see results or if you want to continue challenging yourself, you'll need to change your routine, and you can change it in big ways or small.

You might, for example, add short jogs or faster walks to your walking program to add a little intensity. Or you could try harder poses with your yoga routine, or maybe add a third class each week. Another alternative would be to change your program in a more extreme way, such as taking bike rides rather than walking, or adding a third activity to your program, such as weight training.

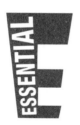

To round out your fitness program, be sure you get plenty of sleep and rest, which means you should take days off and mix up your workouts so that you'll give your body time to recover (remember, muscle gets stronger when you're at rest). And of course, eating well is absolutely a requirement for losing weight (if you need to), and also for having enough energy to get through your workouts.

While you should be very proud of yourself for sticking to a program for six months, that's actually a long time to stay with one program. Your body gets used to a routine in four to eight weeks (depending on your fitness level before you began working out). Now, try to keep in mind that these changes are based on your success as an exerciser, not on any type of failure. Due to homeostasis, the body is resistant to change, which is why it took so much effort to alter both the psychological and physical differences you've achieved. Unfortunately, as a self-regulating machine, once you've achieved those results, the body holds onto this routine and stops making those same steps of progress.

Enjoy Your New Fit Life

This book has given you a lot of information. You might think to yourself, "Hey, I just wanted to walk a little more often!" and that's fine. No one should let the science and facts of why exercise works get in the way of enjoying their favorite activities. The problem, of course, is that many people aren't convinced that exercise is the answer to so many health problems, including obesity, high blood pressure, back pain, heart disease, some cancers, arthritis, depression, and numerous others.

Get Moving!

So, let's say you are now convinced that you want to create a more active life, but you don't want to do it by thinking about heart rate or calorie burning or other scientific elements of exercise. How can you start?

First, create a calendar. Using a calendar is one of the best ways to keep track of your exercise goals and accomplishments on a day-to-day basis. Any old calendar will do, as long as there's enough room to write on it.

Next, ask yourself, "What do I like to do?" or "What do I want to do?" So much of life is "have to," as in, "you have to work" and "you have to pay taxes." It might come as a relief to know that while you *should* exercise, the good news is that you only have to do what you want to do. If you enjoy taking walks, then you can walk. If you enjoy swimming, you can swim. Even gardening can be a form of exercise, as discussed in Chapter 13.

Finally, ask yourself: "How can I turn this into exercise?" As you learned in Chapter 1, a walk or any other activity isn't necessarily exercise if it doesn't get your heart pumping. You need to be sure you are working at a high enough intensity to burn calories, get your heart working harder, and make sure your muscles are being challenged enough so that they'll grow stronger.

So, once you've chosen your activities and made time for them on your calendar, read and understand how to turn a walk—or any other activity—into a workout. That will make all the difference in both your health and your fitness.

Put Together a Complete Plan

It is absolutely true that doing something is better than doing nothing, but it is also absolutely true that the best fitness plans are well-rounded programs and include a variety of activities, including something that gets your heart pumping (walking, jogging, swimming, or biking, for example), something that maintains and builds strength (weight training or yoga), and something that helps you relax in both mind and body (yoga again, as well as Pilates, stretching, and sometimes swimming and other cardio work). Cross-training is far healthier than only doing one form of exercise.

Don't Forget to Have Fun

If, after all of this, you aren't having fun or feeling better, don't give up. Instead, try new activities, try to find active friends to exercise with, and, if necessary, see a doctor and tell her what you've been trying to do and what results you're getting (or not getting). For most of us, fitness feels good whether you're walking more, dancing, or swimming. After all, fitness should make you happy. It's that easy.

Appendix A

Resources

Here are some organizations, magazines, and Web sites that can help you learn more about fitness.

General Information About Health and Fitness

American College of Sports Medicine
www.acsm.org
American Council on Exercise
www.acefitness.org
The Cooper Aerobics Center
www.cooperaerobics.com
Fitday (for workout plans and fitness logs)
www.fitday.com

Magazines

Fitness
www.fitness.com
Men's Health
www.menshealth.com
The New York Times (Tuesday Health section, Thursday Physical Culture page)
www.nytimes.com
Self
www.self.com
Shape
www.shape.com
Prevention
www.prevention.com

Workout Apparel

Adidas
✍www.adidas.com

Asics
✍www.asicsamerica.com

Bike Nashbar
✍www.bikenashbar.com

Champion
✍www.championsports.com

Fleet Feet Sports
✍www.fleetfeet.com

Hind
✍www.hind.com

Insport
✍www.insport.com

New Balance
✍www.newbalance.com

Nike
✍www.nike.com

Pearl Izumi
✍www.Pearlizumi.com

Performance Bicycle
✍www.performancebike.com

Reebok
✍www.reebok.com

Road Runner Sports
✍www.roadrunnersports.com

Women's Apparel

Athleta
✍www.athleta.com

Champion Sports Bras
✍www.championforwomen.com

Moving Comfort
✐*www.movingcomfort.com*
Terry Precision Cycling for Women
✐*www.terrybicycles.com*
Title Nine Sports
✐*www.title9sports.com*

Heart-rate Monitors

Cardiosport
✐*www.cardiosport.com*
Casio
✐*www.casio.com*
Heart Monitors
✐*www.heartmonitor.com*
Heart Zones
✐*www.heartzone.com*
Polar
✐*www.polarusa.com*
Timex Ironman
✐*www.timex.com*

Miscellaneous Equipment

BodyGlide (antichafing petroleum-free lubrication)
✐*www.sternoff.com*
The E3 Grip (Hand grips for body alignment)
✐*www.biogrip.com*
Life Fitness (treadmills)
✐*www.lifefitness.com*
Precor (treadmills)
✐*www.precor.com*
Travelsmith (SPF clothing available)
✐*www.travelsmith.com*

Walkvest

✍*www.walkvest.com*

Swimming

Endless Pools, Inc.

✍*www.endlesspools.com*

Ironman Wetsuits

✍*www.blueseventy.com/ironmanwetsuits*

Speedo

✍*www.speedo.com*

Swimming.com

✍*www.swimming.com*

Tyr

✍*www.tyr.com*

United States Masters Swimming Inc.

✍*www.usms.org*

USA Aquatics

✍*www.usaquatics.com*

Zoggs

✍*www.zoggs.com*

Bicycling

Bicycling.com

✍*www.bicycling.com*

Reebok

✍*www.reebok.com*

Schwinn Cycling and Fitness

✍*www.schwinn.com*

Hands-free Hydration Systems

CamelBak
✍www.camelbak.com

Platypus
✍www.cascadedesigns.com

Ultdir.com
✍www.ultdir.com

Free Weights and Resistance Bands

DynaBand
✍www.fwonline.com

SPRI Products, Inc.
(800) 222-7774

Stretch Cordz—NZ Mfg., Inc.
(800) 886-6621

Tools for Cross-training

Runner's World
✍www.runnersworld.com

Stairmaster Sports Medical Products
✍www.stairmaster.com

The Step Co.
(800) SAY-STEP

Triathlete
✍www.triathletemag.com

Tunturi
✍www.tunturi.com

Exercise Videos

Collage Video
www.collagevideo.com
The Ten-minute Solution DVDs
www.anchorbayentertainment.com
Video Fitness
www.videofitness.com

Gyms

Bally Total Fitness
www.ballyfitness.com
Crunch Fitness
www.crunch.com
YMCA
www.ymca.com

Active Vacations

Abercrombie & Kent
www.abercrombiekent.com
Backroads
www.backroads.com
Learn to Sail
www.offshore-sailing.com
Learn to Surf
www.surfdiva.com or *www.wahinesurfing.com*
Mountain Travel Sobek
www.mtsobek.com
National Geographic Expeditions
www.geox.com
Rails to Trails
www.railstotrails.org

Fitness Spas

Green Valley Spa
✍*www.greenvalleyspa.com*
Mountain Trek Fitness Retreat and Health Spa
✍*www.hiking.com*
Tennessee Fitness Spa
✍*www.tfspa.com*

Sleep Web Sites

American Academy of Sleep Medicine
✍*www.aasmnet.org*
National Sleep Foundation
✍*www.sleepfoundation.org*
Sleepnet.com
✍*www.sleepnet.com*

Nutrition and Eating Organizations

American Dietetic Association
✍*www.eatright.org*
CalorieKing
✍*www.calorieking.com*
Ediets.com
✍*www.ediets.com*
Weight Watchers
✍*www.weightwatchers.com*

Fitness for Kids

KidsHealth
✍*www.kidshealth.org*

LazyTown Entertainment
www.lazytown.com
YMCA
www.ymca.net

Senior Health and Fitness

American Association of Retired Persons
www.aarp.org
Fifty-Plus Lifelong Fitness
www.50plus.org

Appendix B

Workout Plans

No one plan works for everyone, but if you're starting to work out regularly, it's a good idea to write down your plan. First, it helps you visualize and organize what your easy-fitness week is going to look like. Second, it helps you stick with your plans and thus reach your goals, because when something is written down, it seems more official. Here are some blank workout plans organized by activity and goal so you can see the various options you have in creating a workout log for yourself. Remember, too, that there are a number of Web sites as well as books that offer workout logs for all types of activities, fitness levels, and goals. You'll notice that each plan includes space for active intentions so that you can always keep those in mind.

Daily Workout Plan

Active Intentions:

1. _____
2. _____
3. _____

Day	Activity	Time	Intensity	How I Felt
Monday	Walking	45 minutes	Hard	Great! I'm going to do this again on Thursday.
Tuesday				
Wednesday				
Thursday				
Friday				
Saturday				
Sunday				

Cardio Activity Workout Plan

Active Intentions:

1. _____
2. _____
3. _____

Day	Intensity	Distance	Time	How I Felt
Monday				
Tuesday	Easy	2.5 miles	30 minutes	I was a little bored. Should go harder tomorrow
Wednesday				
Thursday				
Friday				
Saturday				
Sunday				

Strength-training Workout Plan

Active Intentions:

1. _____
2. _____
3. _____

Day	Exercise	Weight	Reps/Sets	15/2
Monday				
Tuesday				
Wednesday	Easy	8 lbs.	15/2	Hard. I couldn't finish second set.

Thursday	
Friday	
Saturday	
Sunday	

Workout Plan

Active Intentions:

1. _____
2. _____
3. _____

Sample Exercise Journal

Date: Thursday, October 9

Today I woke up and did five Sun Salutations from my yoga class. It felt really good, and I didn't even have to get out of my pajamas. I had wanted to take a walk at lunch, but I ended up talking to Kate in her office, so, instead, when I left work I took the baby around the block a few times before I cooked dinner. Then before I went to bed, I stretched a little while I watched a *Gilmore Girls* rerun. It felt good. I'm going to lift weights tomorrow.

Sample Eating and Exercise Journal

Active Intentions:

1. _____
2. _____
3. _____

Friday, October 10

- 20-minutes Pilates DVD
- **Breakfast:** Two hard-boiled eggs, glass V-8 juice, one English muffin, 2 tsp. cream cheese, 2 cups coffee with cream.
- **Snack:** Apple, slice of cheddar cheese, two Hershey's kisses.
- **Lunch:** Turkey on rye with lettuce, tomato, mayo, and mustard. Left ¼ of it for tomorrow's morning snack. Banana. Can of soda.
- **Snack:** Two mint cookies, bottle of iced tea.
- **Dinner:** Went to gym and did weights and treadmill for 50 minutes. Salad with lettuce, cucumber, tomato, sprouts, and chicken. No dessert!

Index

THE EVERYTHING SERIES!

BUSINESS & PERSONAL FINANCE

Everything® Accounting Book
Everything® Budgeting Book
Everything® Business Planning Book
Everything® Coaching and Mentoring Book
Everything® Fundraising Book
Everything® Get Out of Debt Book
Everything® Grant Writing Book
Everything® Home-Based Business Book, 2nd Ed.
Everything® Homebuying Book, 2nd Ed.
Everything® Homeselling Book, 2nd Ed.
Everything® Investing Book, 2nd Ed.
Everything® Landlording Book
Everything® Leadership Book
Everything® Managing People Book, 2nd Ed.
Everything® Negotiating Book
Everything® Online Auctions Book
Everything® Online Business Book
Everything® Personal Finance Book
Everything® Personal Finance in Your 20s and 30s Book
Everything® Project Management Book
Everything® Real Estate Investing Book
Everything® Robert's Rules Book, $7.95
Everything® Selling Book
Everything® Start Your Own Business Book, 2nd Ed.
Everything® Wills & Estate Planning Book

COOKING

Everything® Barbecue Cookbook
Everything® Bartender's Book, $9.95
Everything® Chinese Cookbook
Everything® Classic Recipes Book
Everything® Cocktail Parties and Drinks Book
Everything® College Cookbook
Everything® Cooking for Baby and Toddler Book
Everything® Cooking for Two Cookbook
Everything® Diabetes Cookbook
Everything® Easy Gourmet Cookbook
Everything® Fondue Cookbook
Everything® Fondue Party Book
Everything® Gluten-Free Cookbook
Everything® Glycemic Index Cookbook
Everything® Grilling Cookbook

Everything® Healthy Meals in Minutes Cookbook
Everything® Holiday Cookbook
Everything® Indian Cookbook
Everything® Italian Cookbook
Everything® Low-Carb Cookbook
Everything® Low-Fat High-Flavor Cookbook
Everything® Low-Salt Cookbook
Everything® Meals for a Month Cookbook
Everything® Mediterranean Cookbook
Everything® Mexican Cookbook
Everything® One-Pot Cookbook
Everything® Quick and Easy 30-Minute, 5-Ingredient Cookbook
Everything® Quick Meals Cookbook
Everything® Slow Cooker Cookbook
Everything® Slow Cooking for a Crowd Cookbook
Everything® Soup Cookbook
Everything® Tex-Mex Cookbook
Everything® Thai Cookbook
Everything® Vegetarian Cookbook
Everything® Wild Game Cookbook
Everything® Wine Book, 2nd Ed.

GAMES

Everything® 15-Minute Sudoku Book, $9.95
Everything® 30-Minute Sudoku Book, $9.95
Everything® Blackjack Strategy Book
Everything® Brain Strain Book, $9.95
Everything® Bridge Book
Everything® Card Games Book
Everything® Card Tricks Book, $9.95
Everything® Casino Gambling Book, 2nd Ed.
Everything® Chess Basics Book
Everything® Craps Strategy Book
Everything® Crossword and Puzzle Book
Everything® Crossword Challenge Book
Everything® Cryptograms Book, $9.95
Everything® Easy Crosswords Book
Everything® Easy Kakuro Book, $9.95
Everything® Games Book, 2nd Ed.
Everything® Giant Sudoku Book, $9.95
Everything® Kakuro Challenge Book, $9.95
Everything® Large-Print Crossword Challenge Book
Everything® Large-Print Crosswords Book
Everything® Lateral Thinking Puzzles Book, $9.95
Everything® Mazes Book

Everything® Pencil Puzzles Book, $9.95
Everything® Poker Strategy Book
Everything® Pool & Billiards Book
Everything® Test Your IQ Book, $9.95
Everything® Texas Hold 'Em Book, $9.95
Everything® Travel Crosswords Book, $9.95
Everything® Word Games Challenge Book
Everything® Word Search Book

HEALTH

Everything® Alzheimer's Book
Everything® Diabetes Book
Everything® Health Guide to Adult Bipolar Disorder
Everything® Health Guide to Controlling Anxiety
Everything® Health Guide to Fibromyalgia
Everything® Health Guide to Thyroid Disease
Everything® Hypnosis Book
Everything® Low Cholesterol Book
Everything® Massage Book
Everything® Menopause Book
Everything® Nutrition Book
Everything® Reflexology Book
Everything® Stress Management Book

HISTORY

Everything® American Government Book
Everything® American History Book
Everything® Civil War Book
Everything® Freemasons Book
Everything® Irish History & Heritage Book
Everything® Middle East Book

HOBBIES

Everything® Candlemaking Book
Everything® Cartooning Book
Everything® Coin Collecting Book
Everything® Drawing Book
Everything® Family Tree Book, 2nd Ed.
Everything® Knitting Book
Everything® Knots Book
Everything® Photography Book
Everything® Quilting Book
Everything® Scrapbooking Book
Everything® Sewing Book
Everything® Woodworking Book

Bolded titles are new additions to the series.
All Everything® books are priced at $12.95 or $14.95, unless otherwise stated. Prices subject to change without notice.

HOME IMPROVEMENT

Everything® Feng Shui Book
Everything® Feng Shui Decluttering Book, $9.95
Everything® Fix-It Book
Everything® Home Decorating Book
Everything® Home Storage Solutions Book
Everything® Homebuilding Book
Everything® Lawn Care Book
Everything® Organize Your Home Book

KIDS' BOOKS

All titles are $7.95

Everything® Kids' Animal Puzzle & Activity Book
Everything® Kids' Baseball Book, 4th Ed.
Everything® Kids' Bible Trivia Book
Everything® Kids' Bugs Book
Everything® Kids' Cars and Trucks Puzzle & Activity Book
Everything® Kids' Christmas Puzzle & Activity Book
Everything® Kids' Cookbook
Everything® Kids' Crazy Puzzles Book
Everything® Kids' Dinosaurs Book
Everything® Kids' First Spanish Puzzle and Activity Book
Everything® Kids' Gross Hidden Pictures Book
Everything® Kids' Gross Jokes Book
Everything® Kids' Gross Mazes Book
Everything® Kids' Gross Puzzle and Activity Book
Everything® Kids' Halloween Puzzle & Activity Book
Everything® Kids' Hidden Pictures Book
Everything® Kids' Horses Book
Everything® Kids' Joke Book
Everything® Kids' Knock Knock Book
Everything® Kids' Learning Spanish Book
Everything® Kids' Math Puzzles Book
Everything® Kids' Mazes Book
Everything® Kids' Money Book
Everything® Kids' Nature Book
Everything® Kids' Pirates Puzzle and Activity Book
Everything® Kids' Princess Puzzle and Activity Book
Everything® Kids' Puzzle Book
Everything® Kids' Riddles & Brain Teasers Book
Everything® Kids' Science Experiments Book
Everything® Kids' Sharks Book
Everything® Kids' Soccer Book
Everything® Kids' Travel Activity Book

KIDS' STORY BOOKS

Everything® Fairy Tales Book

LANGUAGE

Everything® Conversational Chinese Book with CD, $19.95
Everything® Conversational Japanese Book with CD, $19.95
Everything® French Grammar Book
Everything® French Phrase Book, $9.95
Everything® French Verb Book, $9.95
Everything® German Practice Book with CD, $19.95
Everything® Inglés Book
Everything® Learning French Book
Everything® Learning German Book
Everything® Learning Italian Book
Everything® Learning Latin Book
Everything® Learning Spanish Book
Everything® Russian Practice Book with CD, $19.95
Everything® Sign Language Book
Everything® Spanish Grammar Book
Everything® Spanish Phrase Book, $9.95
Everything® Spanish Practice Book with CD, $19.95
Everything® Spanish Verb Book, $9.95

MUSIC

Everything® Drums Book with CD, $19.95
Everything® Guitar Book
Everything® Guitar Chords Book with CD, $19.95
Everything® Home Recording Book
Everything® Music Theory Book with CD, $19.95
Everything® Reading Music Book with CD, $19.95
Everything® Rock & Blues Guitar Book (with CD), $19.95
Everything® Songwriting Book

NEW AGE

Everything® Astrology Book, 2nd Ed.
Everything® Birthday Personology Book
Everything® Dreams Book, 2nd Ed.
Everything® Love Signs Book, $9.95
Everything® Numerology Book
Everything® Paganism Book
Everything® Palmistry Book
Everything® Psychic Book
Everything® Reiki Book
Everything® Sex Signs Book, $9.95
Everything® Tarot Book, 2nd Ed.
Everything® Wicca and Witchcraft Book

PARENTING

Everything® Baby Names Book, 2nd Ed.
Everything® Baby Shower Book
Everything® Baby's First Food Book
Everything® Baby's First Year Book
Everything® Birthing Book
Everything® Breastfeeding Book
Everything® Father-to-Be Book
Everything® Father's First Year Book
Everything® Get Ready for Baby Book
Everything® Get Your Baby to Sleep Book, $9.95
Everything® Getting Pregnant Book
Everything® Guide to Raising a One-Year-Old
Everything® Guide to Raising a Two-Year-Old
Everything® Homeschooling Book
Everything® Mother's First Year Book
Everything® Parent's Guide to Children and Divorce
Everything® Parent's Guide to Children with ADD/ADHD
Everything® Parent's Guide to Children with Asperger's Syndrome
Everything® Parent's Guide to Children with Autism
Everything® Parent's Guide to Children with Bipolar Disorder
Everything® Parent's Guide to Children with Dyslexia
Everything® Parent's Guide to Positive Discipline
Everything® Parent's Guide to Raising a Successful Child
Everything® Parent's Guide to Raising Boys
Everything® Parent's Guide to Raising Siblings
Everything® Parent's Guide to Sensory Integration Disorder
Everything® Parent's Guide to Tantrums
Everything® Parent's Guide to the Overweight Child
Everything® Parent's Guide to the Strong-Willed Child
Everything® Parenting a Teenager Book
Everything® Potty Training Book, $9.95
Everything® Pregnancy Book, 2nd Ed.
Everything® Pregnancy Fitness Book
Everything® Pregnancy Nutrition Book
Everything® Pregnancy Organizer, 2nd Ed., $16.95
Everything® Toddler Activities Book
Everything® Toddler Book
Everything® Tween Book
Everything® Twins, Triplets, and More Book

PETS

Everything® Aquarium Book
Everything® Boxer Book
Everything® Cat Book, 2nd Ed.
Everything® Chihuahua Book
Everything® Dachshund Book
Everything® Dog Book
Everything® Dog Health Book
Everything® Dog Owner's Organizer, $16.95
Everything® Dog Training and Tricks Book
Everything® German Shepherd Book
Everything® Golden Retriever Book
Everything® Horse Book
Everything® Horse Care Book
Everything® Horseback Riding Book
Everything® Labrador Retriever Book
Everything® Poodle Book
Everything® Pug Book
Everything® Puppy Book
Everything® Rottweiler Book
Everything® Small Dogs Book
Everything® Tropical Fish Book
Everything® Yorkshire Terrier Book

REFERENCE

Everything® Blogging Book
Everything® Build Your Vocabulary Book
Everything® Car Care Book
Everything® Classical Mythology Book
Everything® Da Vinci Book
Everything® Divorce Book
Everything® Einstein Book
Everything® Etiquette Book, 2nd Ed.
Everything® Inventions and Patents Book
Everything® Mafia Book
Everything® Philosophy Book
Everything® Psychology Book
Everything® Shakespeare Book

RELIGION

Everything® Angels Book
Everything® Bible Book
Everything® Buddhism Book
Everything® Catholicism Book
Everything® Christianity Book
Everything® History of the Bible Book
Everything® Jesus Book
Everything® Jewish History & Heritage Book
Everything® Judaism Book
Everything® Kabbalah Book
Everything® Koran Book
Everything® Mary Book

Everything® Mary Magdalene Book
Everything® Prayer Book
Everything® Saints Book
Everything® Torah Book
Everything® Understanding Islam Book
Everything® World's Religions Book
Everything® Zen Book

SCHOOL & CAREERS

Everything® Alternative Careers Book
Everything® Career Tests Book
Everything® College Major Test Book
Everything® College Survival Book, 2nd Ed.
Everything® Cover Letter Book, 2nd Ed.
Everything® Filmmaking Book
Everything® Get-a-Job Book
Everything® Guide to Being a Paralegal
Everything® Guide to Being a Real Estate Agent
Everything® Guide to Being a Sales Rep
Everything® Guide to Careers in Health Care
Everything® Guide to Careers in Law Enforcement
Everything® Guide to Government Jobs
Everything® Guide to Starting and Running a Restaurant
Everything® Job Interview Book
Everything® New Nurse Book
Everything® New Teacher Book
Everything® Paying for College Book
Everything® Practice Interview Book
Everything® Resume Book, 2nd Ed.
Everything® Study Book

SELF-HELP

Everything® Dating Book, 2nd Ed.
Everything® Great Sex Book
Everything® Kama Sutra Book
Everything® Self-Esteem Book

SPORTS & FITNESS

Everything® Easy Fitness Book
Everything® Fishing Book
Everything® Golf Instruction Book
Everything® Pilates Book
Everything® Running Book
Everything® Weight Training Book
Everything® Yoga Book

TRAVEL

Everything® Family Guide to Cruise Vacations
Everything® Family Guide to Hawaii

Everything® Family Guide to Las Vegas, 2nd Ed.
Everything® Family Guide to Mexico
Everything® Family Guide to New York City, 2nd Ed.
Everything® Family Guide to RV Travel & Campgrounds
Everything® Family Guide to the Caribbean
Everything® Family Guide to the Walt Disney World Resort®, Universal Studios®, and Greater Orlando, 4th Ed.
Everything® Family Guide to Timeshares
Everything® Family Guide to Washington D.C., 2nd Ed.
Everything® Guide to New England

WEDDINGS

Everything® Bachelorette Party Book, $9.95
Everything® Bridesmaid Book, $9.95
Everything® Destination Wedding Book
Everything® Elopement Book, $9.95
Everything® Father of the Bride Book, $9.95
Everything® Groom Book, $9.95
Everything® Mother of the Bride Book, $9.95
Everything® Outdoor Wedding Book
Everything® Wedding Book, 3rd Ed.
Everything® Wedding Checklist, $9.95
Everything® Wedding Etiquette Book, $9.95
Everything® Wedding Organizer, 2nd Ed., $16.95
Everything® Wedding Shower Book, $9.95
Everything® Wedding Vows Book, $9.95
Everything® Wedding Workout Book
Everything® Weddings on a Budget Book, $9.95

WRITING

Everything® Creative Writing Book
Everything® Get Published Book, 2nd Ed.
Everything® Grammar and Style Book
Everything® Guide to Writing a Book Proposal
Everything® Guide to Writing a Novel
Everything® Guide to Writing Children's Books
Everything® Guide to Writing Research Papers
Everything® Screenwriting Book
Everything® Writing Poetry Book
Everything® Writing Well Book

Available wherever books are sold!
To order, call 800-258-0929, or visit us at *www.everything.com*
Everything® and everything.com® are registered trademarks of F+W Publications, Inc.

10

George and Marie
Loribond

14. 9. 44.